"*The Healthy Gut Workbook* is extremely informative and easy to follow. It's a must-read for everyone who wants to improve not only their gut health, but their overall health as well."

—Adam Perlman, MD, MPH, FACP, UMDNJ Endowed Professor of Complementary and Alternative Medicine at the University of Medicine and Dentistry of New Jersey

"From one of America's master teachers and an authority on integrative health, Victor Sierpina, *The Healthy Gut Workbook* is one of the most accurate and concise guidebooks on gastrointestinal health to appear in years. Filled with good science and good sense, this book takes the mystery out of functional integrative medicine, one of the most important approaches to health of the past decade. Let Dr. Sierpina be your guide to superb gastrointestinal health!"

—Larry Dossey, MD, author of *The Power of Premonitions*

"Dr. Sierpina, one of the nation's most respected integrative medicine experts, has done all patients with bowel problems a huge favor by writing this clear, simple, and accessible manual outlining the most important elements they need to know to take charge of their health. His extensive clinical experience and very user-friendly writing style make this self-assessment tool a pleasure to use. An important contribution to patient literature on bowel dysfunction."

—Woodson Merrell, MD, assistant Clinical Professor of Medicine at Columbia Medical School and author of *Power Up*

THE
HEALTHY GUT WORKBOOK

WHOLE-BODY HEALING FOR HEARTBURN, ULCERS, CONSTIPATION, IBS, DIVERTICULOSIS & MORE

VICTOR S. SIERPINA, MD

New Harbinger Publications, Inc.

Publisher's Note

This publication is designed to provide accurate and authoritative information in regard to the subject matter covered. It is sold with the understanding that the publisher is not engaged in rendering psychological, financial, legal, or other professional services. If expert assistance or counseling is needed, the services of a competent professional should be sought.

Distributed in Canada by Raincoast Books

Copyright © 2010 by Victor S. Sierpina
New Harbinger Publications, Inc.
5674 Shattuck Avenue
Oakland, CA 94609
www.newharbinger.com

Acquired by Jess O'Brien; Cover design by Sara Christian; Edited by Brady Kahn

FSC
Mixed Sources
Product group from well-managed
forests and other controlled sources
Cert no. SW-COC-002283
www.fsc.org
© 1996 Forest Stewardship Council

RAINFOREST ALLIANCE CERTIFIED

Library of Congress Cataloging-in-Publication Data

Sierpina, Victor S., 1949-
  The healthy gut workbook : whole-body healing for heartburn, ulcers, constipation, IBS, diverticulosis, and more / Victor S. Sierpina.
     p. cm.
  Includes bibliographical references and index.
  ISBN 978-1-57224-844-1
  1. Gastrointestinal system--Diseases--Alternative treatment--Popular works. 2. Naturopathy--Popular works. I. Title.
  RC806.S55 2010
  616.3'06--dc22

                    2010025531

12 11 10   10 9 8 7 6 5 4 3 2 1   First printing

CONTENTS

PART 1
THE HEALTHY GUT

PART 2
SOME THINGS YOU CAN DO FOR YOUR GUT

FOREWORD

The Healthy Gut Workbook will prove to be an important publication that adds to the expanding body of literature about functional integrative medicine.

Functional medicine is a systems-medicine approach that addresses the primary challenge of the twentieth century: improving prevention and treatment for complex, chronic illness. These textbooks together set the boundaries, evidence, and methodologies for providing a new, comprehensive, clinically relevant medical paradigm shift for achieving this urgent goal.

What is the real importance, you may ask, of functional medicine and, in particular, of this latest publication, *The Healthy Gut Workbook*, based on the application of functional medicine? We currently have in place in the industrialized world a method of health care developed and based on the twentieth-century acute-care medical model. Such a model is characterized by rapid differential diagnosis—with an organ-systems focus—aimed at prescribing a drug (or procedure) that will ameliorate the patient's presenting symptoms and avert the immediate threat. It is a model that evolved in response to the primary causes of morbidity and mortality in the last century, namely acute infections and trauma. The experts, you will recognize, within this organ-systems model are the various specialists within conventional medicine, such as gastroenterologists, cardiologists, pulmonologists, endocrinologists, neurologists, and orthopaedic surgeons.

Inherently, this acute-care methodology minimizes the involvement of the patient, who functions mostly as a passive recipient of the procedure or prescription. It prioritizes immediate solutions to the most pressing problems. It is, of course, absolutely essential in emergency and hospital-based care of many kinds, but difficulties arise when this model is applied to ongoing, community-based care for the nonacute, chronic conditions that represent 80 percent of the daily work of present-day clinicians (Holman 2004).

The Healthy Gut Workbook takes the principles of functional medicine and shows how they can be usefully applied by those most in need: people with symptoms and signs involving the health of the gastrointestinal tract. In so doing, it illustrates the shift that will be required to enfold into twentieth-century medical practice the innovative clinical practices of patient-centered, personalized, systems-based medicine.

Clinical decision making, when exercised at the most efficacious level, drills deeply into the "why" of every diagnosis. Pursuit of the elusive network of causality in the deeper intersections of genetic individuality, within each client's unique context of living, is an essential responsibility of the clinician. However, this clinical workbook illustrates, using step-by-step examples, how to achieve more satisfying outcomes through easy-to-understand treatment programs that can be followed by the layperson. The author shows you how to take back your digestive health without the need for skills learned through rigorous training in functional medicine. He has done the hard work of understanding the essential components for achieving digestive health and makes specific efficacious interventions easily available to the reader.

Hence, *The Healthy Gut Workbook* will prove to be an important publication about functional and integrative medicine in clinical practice with a focus on gastrointestinal health. I hope you enjoy the discussions and practical applications herein, as they so well exemplify the clinical application of this important medical model. I hope that this innovative workbook encourages a series of patient-friendly how-to workbooks that assist those living with complex chronic health issues to achieve the health and wellness they deserve.

—David S. Jones, MD, FABFP
    President of the Institute for Functional Medicine
    Director of Medical Education, IFM

PREFACE

Well before the end of the first decade of life, virtually every person has had multiple episodes of gastrointestinal "memorable events." In fact, on a daily basis, the all-important gut makes sure we experience the sounds, smells, and rumbles of this key player in the quest for a lifetime of super health. This is quite unique in that we don't take notice of many other body parts unless they hurt or malfunction in some obvious way.

Gastrointestinal health begins no later than birth, when vaginal delivery sets the stage for each person's unique set of gut bacteria. In most cases, breastfeeding soon follows. Breast milk not only supplies all the nutrients for the newborn infant, but also contains so-called prebiotics, which supply nourishment that promotes the growth of healthy probiotic bacteria. So, pick your mom carefully, as the quest for a twenty-first-century super gut begins soon after leaving mom's birth canal.

When I wrote the SuperFoods Rx series of books, I initially did a thorough review of the nutrients associated with enhanced longevity. I then found the superfoods that contained these remarkable health-promoting substances. Although all organ systems are essential, it all starts with the gut. If we are unable to digest and absorb fats, proteins, carbohydrates, certain parts of fiber, vitamins, minerals, and phytonutrients, poor health is soon to follow. Every cell in the body is dependent on nutrients processed in the gastrointestinal tract.

One key to successful aging is to eat a more nutrient dense (superfood) diet. Like every other organ system function, maturity is eventually associated with diminished efficiency. When it comes to the gut, this means fewer nutrients extracted and absorbed from our meals. As a result, we must increasingly eat a nutrient dense, for the most part calorie sparse, high-fiber superfood diet. Another important factor is that at least 70 percent of our entire immune system, the so-called GALT (gut-associated lymphoid tissue), is located in our gastrointestinal tract. I always tell my patients to be kind to their immune system if they want to achieve super health. What I am really saying is to be kind to your gut, because this sets the stage for controlling not only overall immune system vitality, but body-wide inflammation as well. And remember, inflammation is the harbinger for the later development of poor health and the onset of virtually every disease known to modern man.

A healthy gut is a great example of how multiple lifestyle and food choices work in synergy to promote health. Physical activity, stress and anxiety reduction, sleep, superfoods, fiber, spices (including turmeric, black pepper, and ginger), portion control, probiotic bacteria, and foods containing prebiotic "food" for health-promoting gut bacteria (such as green tea, honey, whole grains, blueberries, and breast milk) all work together to promote gastrointestinal and body-wide health. With 70 percent of Americans now overweight or obese, preliminary but quite convincing scientific studies suggest that our gut bacteria play an important role in processing calories in such a way as to contribute to the worldwide obesity epidemic. The gut bacteria found in those eating a highly processed, non-superfood diet (the majority of Americans) very efficiently process these calories into excess body weight. On the other hand, the gut bacterial flora found in those eating a superfood type diet are rather stingy in providing excess calories to our body.

I want to congratulate my good friend, Dr. Vic Sierpina, for writing *The Healthy Gut Workbook*. This must-read for everyone interested in achieving a twenty-first-century super gut gives the reader a clear, practical, and science-based program to implement in daily life. Roll up your sleeves and get ready to work your way through Dr. Vic's quizzes. I found them very informative and useful. After reading this outstanding addition to understanding all aspects of gut health, the reader will have an easy-to-follow action plan for optimizing this all-important thirty feet of the body.

—Steven G. Pratt, MD

ACKNOWLEDGMENTS

First, I want to thank my wife, Michelle Sierpina, Ph.D., for her invaluable assistance in bringing birth to this book. She has been there since its early conception to help nurture and feed it through the nearly yearlong incubation period. She has been a midwife to chapter rewrites, resources, and improving my choice of words, metaphors, and humor. She also has set aside a good number of personal and family duties or taken on ones I should have been doing during this long birthing process. For all this, I thank her immensely.

I could not have achieved much of the richness and depth of the book without the wisdom of my colleagues and teachers at the Institute for Functional Medicine (IFM). David Jones, Patrick Hanaway, Jerry Mullin, Liz Lipski, Joe Lamb, and, of course, Jeff Bland are a few of the many from that excellent learning organization that I could name. Their continual research, clinical practice, and teaching have informed the new model of systems biology called *functional medicine*.

Their willingness to generously share with me the developed resources, worksheets, and other materials from IFM programs and publications helps get functional medicine to the world.

Steve Pratt is a "super Doc" whose SuperFood approach to life has long energized me and my family, students, and patients. His hard work and research have helped shape many aspects of this book. Brittanya Washington's cool, competent computer skills in assembling and formatting resources were critical to bringing the book to completion on time.

And finally I appreciate the professionalism and teamwork at New Harbinger in helping to bring this book to the public. Jess O'Brien, Wendy Millstine, and Jess Beebe worked closely with my literary agent Barbara Deal and me through all stages of the book's initial growth and development to bring it to you for your improved health. Thanks, too, to Brady Kahn for her patient, thoughtful editing and for dealing with my occasional conniption fits.

Thanks to you all.

INTRODUCTION

Gastrointestinal (GI) problems affect all of the people some of the time and some of the people all of the time. Indeed, GI problems are one of our most common afflictions. Since you are reading this book, my guess is that you or someone close to you has a digestive problem that you would like to improve. This workbook offers many tools and techniques to do just that.

A few years ago, I was doing research for a medical mission group to determine the most common botanical medicines used in the area of Nicaragua where the group was planning to go. Many indigenous plants were used as home remedies there, as they are throughout many countries in the world. I was astonished that so many of these remedies were for gastrointestinal complaints, from worms and parasites to diarrhea, gas, constipation, ulcers, and liver problems. The number of concoctions listed for GI problems exceeded any other physical category.

This emphasized for me that what I have observed in over thirty years of primary care practice is true. Bellyaches and GI problems are extremely common everywhere. The kinds of conditions seen in underdeveloped countries may be somewhat different from what we experience in places like the United States, but digestive problems are a major health issue the world over. Indeed, I have researched a vast number of therapeutic approaches for GI issues in other systems of medicine representing the people and cultures of India, China, the Caribbean, Latin America, and Africa.

Many GI problems that bring people to the modern medical doctor or traditional healer are short-term and self-limited. These include problems like stomach flu, nausea, vomiting, diarrhea, indigestion, gas, constipation, and infantile colic. Others are troubling chronic conditions such as heartburn, inflammatory bowel disease, irritable bowel disease, malabsorption, and gallstones, as well as certain liver and pancreatic conditions.

The approach I take in this workbook is a holistic one. It is integrative in bringing together evidence-based modern medical treatments with traditional, natural, and complementary remedies. I emphasize not only treatment but also prevention through sound nutrition and a balanced lifestyle.

Further, my approach is ecologically sound "green medicine," a systems-biology approach known as *functional medicine*. This approach does not merely define medical issues in terms of certain disease states or specific organ dysfunctions, but rather it incorporates an integrative view of how all body systems and the gut interact. It is becoming well known that an ecological model is the best solution to many of the planet's problems. Everything is in some way connected to everything else. It is the same in your body.

How and what you eat is due not only to your food choices but also to the conditions of soil and sea, agricultural and fishing practices, pesticides and toxins in the environment, culture, cooking methods, and food availability. These ecological and global factors affect our health and that of our world community's most vulnerable, including infants and the frail elderly.

Getting relief from chronic, complex medical conditions, including those of the GI system, requires such a holistic and ecological viewpoint. An example of a functional-medicine approach is as follows. Have you, or has someone you know, ever felt vaguely sick, achy, fatigued, or just "blah?" If you brought those general complaints to your doctor, he or she might not find any specific problem, such as an infection, ulcer, or other explanation, despite thorough examination and testing. The functional-medicine approach helps in this situation by identifying conditions that affect *function* even before they can be characterized as a medical condition. So the fatigued and "blah" feeling might be due to a food allergy, chronic inflammation, or gut bacterial imbalance that wouldn't show up in regular blood or X-ray tests but can nevertheless affect how you are feeling and functioning day to day.

The gut is the conduit of good health and poor health. If misused, it can contribute to many illnesses far removed from the abdominal cavity. Poor nutrition leads, of course, to obesity and its attendant problems. These include risk factors responsible for the epidemic of childhood diabetes, osteoarthritis, high cholesterol, peripheral vascular and cardiovascular disease, and hypertension. Food sensitivities and allergies also contribute to many of these diseases by stimulating chronic, silent inflammation. Such inflammation wreaks its damage by depressing the immune system, which leads to recurrent infections such as those of the sinuses, respiratory tract, skin, and other structures.

This workbook's functional, ecological approach is based first in your personal story. I encourage you to understand your own story of both illness and wellness through a number of exercises, including diet and symptom diaries. The stories of others included in this book may remind you of your own problems or those of friends and family members. This book offers approaches to the most common GI problems. It examines the interaction of these problems with all aspects of health and includes helpful tables listing the full range of therapeutic options.

Your story and history are vital, since the underlying causes of disease are complex and often deeply rooted. All of the following can play a significant role in your GI health and wellness: genetics, physical and psychological trauma, sexuality, environmental issues, stress, relationships, sleep patterns, diet, exercise, spiritual perspective, use of medications, and exposure to toxins. Without an understanding of the influences of these factors on the terrain of your health, we may miss important turning points or conditions that led to your being prone to acquire a particular condition. These factors also may have triggered your disease or continue to sustain and aggravate your gut condition.

After reading this book, you will have some important self-assessment tools for your own GI health that hopefully will expand beyond how you have thought about it previously. A number of exercises and worksheets will help you assess your lifestyle, behaviors, and health risks, showing you how these impact your gut health and overall well-being.

Included are methods for identifying food sensitivities and allergies, as well as several specialized diets to help you improve your gut health. This book will also help you weigh the benefits and risks of using certain GI medications.

I hope you enjoy the positive approach taken to creating a healthier diet and lifestyle. Practical tips include a list of SuperFoods and behavioral change methods that will help you heal your gut and your life. Eating well, managing stress, exercising, and cultivating a mindful movement practice can all contribute to a healthier gut and a healthier life in mind-body and spirit. This allows you to enjoy the fruit of your talents, time with family and friends, and rewarding work, all without being impaired by poor gut health, belly pain, and the limitations of various preventable gut-related illnesses.

A NOTE OF CAUTION

I strongly support self-care, personal health empowerment, and improving your understanding of gut health. However, these cannot substitute for evaluation by a trained health professional in cases of long-standing or undiagnosed symptoms. This book is thus not meant as a substitute for professional medical judgment, though it can serve as a helpful adjunct to it.

When in doubt about your digestive health, see your doctor or other health professional to exclude serious and potentially life-threatening conditions, like cancer, infections, inflammatory conditions, stones, and bleeding. Problems such as these may lie hidden and out of your sight or understanding within the abdominal cavity. Be safe, be sane, be healthy.

Get a complete history and exam from a reliable practitioner if you have any question as to what is going on inside your abdomen. In some cases, this will require blood, urine, or stool testing, imaging studies, or endoscopic procedures. Regular screening with colonoscopy for those at high risk and those over fifty can save lives through early detection and treatment of colon polyps and cancers. Immunizations can reduce risk of serious diarrhea and hepatitis. In a word, be kind to yourself and your belly. Do what you can within the boundaries of common sense and good hygiene to keep well and attend to acute, self-limiting conditions. Seek medical attention for longer-standing problems and be willing to try an expanded range of therapeutic options as described here if standard medical therapy is not offering complete relief.

PART 1

THE HEALTHY GUT

CHAPTER 1

YOUR GUT

AN OWNER'S MANUAL

As owner and operator of the food tube called the gut, wouldn't you like to have a better understanding of its component parts and how they work together? This chapter provides a description of gut processes and plumbing. It is a brief overview of digestive system anatomy and physiology for you, the informed consumer of food and beverages. While many medical texts cover this topic in depth, I will give you enough information, as briefly as possible, to make the rest of the book understandable and usable.

As you travel through the chapters ahead and do the various exercises, you'll be well on your way to a healthy gut. In this spirit, I offer an ode of appreciation to the gut. It gives perspective to the overall value of nutrition and the gastrointestinal (GI) system to your life.

ODE TO THE GUT

Like the late comedian Rodney Dangerfield, the gut gets no respect. Its value in medicine and culture is far overshadowed by such organs as the heart, the eye, and the brain. Even Chinese medicine, which calls the heart the "emperor of organs," gives a much stronger emphasis to the kidney than to the earthy elements in the gut.

A verse from the Good Book (1 Corinthians 12–26) reminds us that each part of the body is vital and no part should be disrespected. Yet the gut, with its often embarrassing rumblings, outgassings, burps, belches, flatulence, vomitus, and olfactorily offensive offal is a bit like the slightly demented aunt, best kept quietly out of sight and out of discussion. This is an egregious error of epic proportions!

For example, consider the merits of the anus. First, remember the anus is the other end of a kiss. The sumptuous, sensuous lips are at the head of the river of intake to the gut. Lips are prominently featured in magazines, fashion photos, and the like. Alas, the poor anus remains hidden and uncelebrated. Yet get a pain in the a … (nus), and note how quickly it is noticed in the brain. What other muscle in the body has such versatility and refined control? A true super muscle, it is able to contain and selectively eliminate gas, liquid, or solid matter! In these functions, it far exceeds the potential of the hand, our most developed tool-holding member.

Such a monstrous injustice! What body part was likely mentioned the last time you heard someone being spoken of disparagingly? This puts the excellent and essential anus in further disrepute. The anus sadly can draw little comfort from the fact that its urogenital neighbors also get lumped into such expletives and vituperatives. In any case, I call for nothing less than a revolution for gut appreciation.

In this brave new world of respect for the gut, the GI tract will be returned to its rightful place as the "river of life." Like the Colorado, the Rio Grande, the Nile, or other great rivers, life without a gut is unimaginable.

We may abuse the gut with fast and fatty food, too much or too little food, toxins, and other misdemeanors and felonies, but remember that good health and good immunity begin with healthy nutrition and a healthy gut. Life itself is dependent on this lowly, gurgling, smelly organ system, without which the magnificent galaxy of other organs could not long endure.

So now … pucker up as if preparing to give a kiss and project loving energy to your gut, from stem to stern, from the beginning of the kiss to its end.

GROSS ANATOMY: THE SHORT COURSE

We start by taking a tour of the gut from start to finish. A general diagram of the GI tract is included for easy reference (see figure 1).

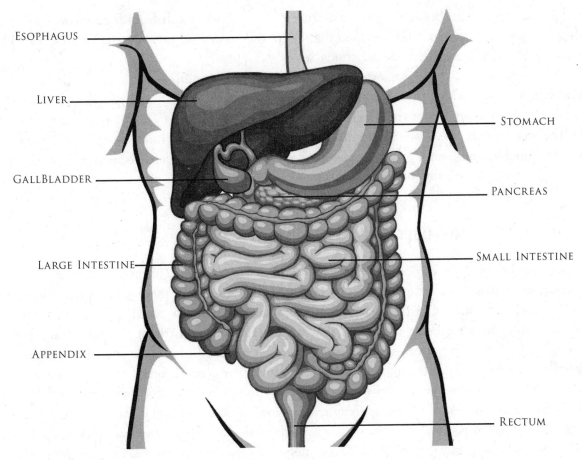

ESOPHAGUS

LIVER

GALLBLADDER

LARGE INTESTINE

APPENDIX

STOMACH

PANCREAS

SMALL INTESTINE

RECTUM

FIGURE 1: DIAGRAM OF THE DIGESTIVE TRACT

Oral Beginnings: Lips, Tongue, Mouth, Throat

The beginning of the GI tract anatomically is the lips, mouth, tongue, and *pharynx* (throat). Imagine biting into a bright-yellow sour lemon. Notice the pucker and saliva in your mouth. Now you realize that the functions of the mouth begin elsewhere in the brain, in the *cephalic*, or head phase, of digestion. Even thinking about and smelling the aromas from Mama's kitchen or a fine restaurant will start saliva and other digestive juices flowing—before you've taken one bite. This process of digestion is beyond the mechanical acts of biting and chewing or the simple tastes of sweet, sour, salty, or spicy. It is a complex dance between thoughts, experiences, expectations, and the world of food and drink. Any good wine connoisseur knows that the nose and the subtle scents it can detect are as vital a part of the tasting experience as what happens in the mouth. This is protective to our health, since we can detect with high degrees of sensitivity when food is spoiled or offensive and therefore likely to make us sick. The salivary glands help to lubricate our food as we chew it and begin the digestive process. As you may recall from high school biology, saliva contains an enzyme called *amylase* that starts the process of breaking down starches and carbohydrates well before they hit the stomach.

Once a mouthful of food is chewed, moistened with saliva, and ready to swallow, the muscles of *deglutition* (swallowing) go to work. These, in the back of the mouth and pharynx, are orchestrated with the movements of the tongue, the closing of the opening to the airway, the *epiglottis*, and the relaxation of the *upper esophageal sphincter*. This area, rich in immune cells, includes the tonsils, adenoids, and lymph glands in the neck and acts as a major defense against bacteria and viruses, keeping them from entering your system.

Heading Downstream: Esophagus

The swallowing, or deglutition process, starts the *bolus*—the lump of chewed food—downstream toward the stomach, moving it from the pharynx. From there it is carried down the *esophagus*, a tube connecting the mouth to the stomach, through a coordinated process called *peristalsis*. Imagine a pig being swallowed slowly by a large boa constrictor. The unfortunate pig moves along the boa's intestine as a progressively smaller bolus as it becomes dinner for the beast. Peristalsis is similar, basically a progressive series of muscular contractions propelling food to the lower esophagus, where another valve relaxes and lets food enter the stomach. Later you'll hear about this valve, the *lower esophageal sphincter*. It allows food to enter the stomach and prevents food from backing up from the stomach. Exceptions to this are *reverse peristalsis*, normally called vomiting, and *gastroesophageal reflux* (GERD), reflux of food and stomach acids into the esophagus. The esophagus is lined with mucus-secreting glands to protect it from such acid baths.

A Churning, Squeezing, Acid Bath: Stomach

The stomach, a muscular organ about the size of a football, is an amazing part of the GI system. The inside is covered with thick folds called *rugae*, allowing expansion and contraction, mixing and mashing of food. The acidity level in the stomach would burn a hole in your skin if applied undiluted, yet the stomach secretes these powerful acids and, in the healthy state, is protected by its lining and various mucus secretions against dissolving itself. This acid kills bacteria and is important in protecting against infections and helping absorption of various nutrients and micronutrients.

Once food enters the stomach, it is temporarily stored there. Acid secretion is stimulated while a wide variety of other chemicals and enzymes needed for digestion are called into action downstream. The stomach is a complex signal transmitter along with the *duodenum*, the outlet of the stomach into the small intestine.

In the stomach, powerful muscles churn food as it starts to turn from solid to a semi-solid or liquid consistency called *chyme*. From there, it continues its peristaltic-driven journey through the bowels. Complex chemical reactions are initiated, giving signals to coordinate digestion. All this happens under the control of the *autonomic nervous system*, largely independent of conscious control.

Only a few substances are absorbed directly from the stomach; these include water, alcohol, and aspirin. The vast majority of absorption of food, liquids, and nutrients occurs in the small intestine.

Absorbing and More: Small Intestine

The small intestine is about twenty-five to thirty feet long in the average adult. If the absorptive surface of the small intestine, composed of many folds of tissue, were unfolded, it would cover the area of a doubles tennis court. It is in this zone that the essential nutrients from food and drink are absorbed. The small intestine is composed of three parts: the *duodenum*, *jejunum*, and *ileum*. Those many folds help absorb fluid and nutrients and are home to the largest collection of immune tissue in the body. These cells, called *Peyer's patches*, constitute the gut's function as a major player in our immune system. This tissue is also called GALT (gut-associated lymphoid tissue).

Digestive juices stimulate hormones like *cholecystokinin*, which causes the gallbladder to contract and secrete bile stored from the liver into the small intestine. Bile then starts to digest and emulsify fats. The pancreas secretes powerful digestive enzymes, such as lipase, amylase, and peptidases, to help break down fats, carbohydrates, and proteins into smaller and more absorbable elements. Bicarbonate ions from the pancreas and bile from the liver help neutralize the intense acidity of the stomach acids so these other digestive processes can occur.

By now, food particles have been broken down into more elemental parts: carbohydrates into starches and simple sugars, proteins into peptides gand amino acids, fats into smaller lipid particles like triglycerides and cholesterol. With help from additional enzymes in the small intestinal lining, these all cross the membranes of the small intestine and are absorbed into the bloodstream. They then travel to the liver where they are processed and subjected to further biochemical degradation, detoxification, and processing. The liver, the biochemical factory of the body, is home to thousands of chemical reactions, all of which are essential to completing the work of utilizing food. From the liver, these nutrients enter our bloodstream and cells. Meanwhile, back in the small intestine, the remnants of food are entering the *ileum*. This is the last part of the small intestine, emptying into the portion of the colon called the *cecum* where the *appendix*, which is chock-full of immune cells, is attached. The appendix can become inflamed, causing a surgical emergency; it also serves as another part of the immune system to protect us from infections going through the gut.

Water Treatment Plant: Colon

The *colon*, or large intestine, shaped like an inverted U, starts in the right lower part of our belly at the cecum and appendix, and becomes the *ascending colon, transverse colon, descending colon, sigmoid colon, rectum,* and *anus.*

Most of us think of the colon as the place where waste from digestion is processed and eliminated, but the colon does even more. It is like a city's water treatment plant. The colon receives the chyme from the small intestine and then extracts large amounts of water, along with vitamins, minerals, and other nutrients. It gradually compacts this material into the solid waste of indigestible fiber and other waste matter that becomes your stool. In doing so, one of the major functions of the colon is to reabsorb large quantities of water from the stool. For an idea of the amount of water involved, consider a bad case of diarrhea and how much fluid the colon excretes when it isn't absorbing water normally. Diseases like cholera, which interfere with water absorption in the colon, can cause such severe diarrhea (several gallons a day) that they may lead to dehydration and death. The colon is home to billions of bacteria that are vital to your health as it compresses and regulates extraction of fluid from your waste matter. Once the colon has condensed the remains of your digestion, it moves this fecal mass into the sigmoid colon and rectum. When these portions of the colon are distended, nerve fibers send a signal to your brain encouraging release of the stool through the anal sphincter. This process is voluntary through most of our lives, except during infancy and sometimes illness or old age. This final process, defecation, is as important to your health as the food you place in your mouth. Strained, irregular, or too frequent stools can create major problems in your health and your experience of wellness.

Maintaining a healthy in-and-out flow, like the ancient Chinese philosophical concept of *yin* and *yang,* is key to keeping a happy and healthy gut. It also leads to the optimal well-being of other organ systems.

CONCLUSION

As you can tell from this brief journey through the gut, the process of digestion is almost entirely automatic, highly complex, and one of nature's true miracles. There are many places along this river of life in which the process of digestion can malfunction. Some problems that can occur are inflammation, too much or too little acid, things flowing backward instead of forward, peristalsis that is too fast or too slow, imbalances in chemical factories like the liver and pancreas, infections, tumors, stones, problems with blood flow, blockages, growths, hernias, structural abnormalities, and trauma. There are also many ways that you can help these conditions improve or, better yet, prevent them from occurring. That is the subject of the rest of this workbook.

In the meantime, let's eat.

CHAPTER 2

FOOD, GLORIOUS FOOD!

THE JOYS OF EATING HEALTHFULLY

To find our best health zone, to enjoy our food socially, ethnically, and from a culinary dimension, we must rid ourselves of both overconsumption and the guilt that accompanies it.

Food is a glorious, essential ingredient to a healthy life. In every culture, in every society, food is a central ingredient of daily life, major celebrations, and religious rituals. It is and should be a source of fun, socialization, cultural normality, family time, and more. For human beings, there is something entirely primeval about food. Without it, we die. With it, we live and have the potential to prosper. Life without the enjoyment of food is unimaginable and impossible. So let's take a look at food throughout history and how we can better enjoy our life through healthful eating and a balanced lifestyle.

A SHORT HISTORY OF FOOD

Orphans in Victorian England, as told in Dickens's novel *Oliver Twist*, were fed a thin gruel of water and mashed grain. This gruel kept the poor orphans alive, barely. Dickens used this staple of the poorhouse as a symbol of cruelty, deprivation, and starvation. In the musical version of the story, the orphans sing about all the "food, glorious food" that's missing from their diet: meat, bread, desserts, fruits, and more.

Average heights, as well as neurological development, of children in most countries have increased substantially since the Victorian era as nutrition for children has improved over the gruel level. Feeding children adequate amounts of a mixture of healthy proteins, fats, and carbohydrates has eliminated the scourges of rickets, beriberi, pellagra, scurvy, and other kinds of malnutrition. In some parts of the world, an obesity problem has replaced a famine problem.

In the American society where I live and practice medicine, starvation is rarely a reality in terms of health risk. This is not to minimize that some poor children, adults, and senior citizens lack access to and budget for quality food. They may ingest adequate calories that are unfortunately overloaded with refined carbohydrates and fats and contain minimal fruits and vegetables.

Too often in our society, excess calories lead to health problems. Childhood obesity and associated diseases like diabetes are an epidemic threatening the health of young people and that of future generations. Can you imagine kids of today getting cardiac stents and other medical procedures for diabetic complications in their twenties and thirties? It is a significant risk and a potential huge financial burden to society.

Recent movies and books like *Supersize Me*, *Fast Food Nation*, and *Food, Inc.* highlight the dangers of oversupplying calories to both adults and children, particularly foods that are high in fat, low in fiber, with a *high glycemic index*. These are foods such as refined carbohydrates that convert quickly to sugar in our bodies.

The challenge is that we haven't always had it so good. Historically, periods of feast alternated with periods of famine. Accumulating a bank account of fat might ensure survival during leaner, colder, and hungrier times. Being too thin as a child or an adult put one much closer to starvation. I still remember my old-country Polish grandmother, whose folk attitude was "fat baby—good!" In her day, a scrawny child was less likely to survive a case of pneumonia, diarrhea, or any other common disease or even a long winter. So my Babcia had it right. She died fat (er ... stocky) and happy at ninety-four years old.

Yet many people in our society who are trying to lose weight come up against the metabolic wall that this genetic history has created as an adaptive survival mechanism. Starve yourself and your metabolism slows down. Feed it more than it needs, and it's like money in the bank to store or even hoard. We then surround this human bank vault of fat, calories, and memories of plentiful times with metabolic and psychological walls that keep us from allowing excess weight to drop away. Add an inactive lifestyle, and you have a genetic and societal recipe for obesity.

Those ancient cave dwellers, nomads, and farmers had to move around a lot and work really hard to catch, find, and grow their food. I think about my grandparents, my parents, and other relatives who made our traditional Polish dishes a focal point of holidays, family gatherings, and cultural identity. The same is true of many immigrants, whether from India, Latin America, Italy, or Iraq. Each group is held together by a bond of family, shared history, and a communal menu of ethnic foods.

Our American ethnic traditions have many wonderful and healthy foods, often derived from pioneering and rural lives. A healthy, active farmer like my grandfather, or my father, who worked as a heavy equipment mechanic, could easily gobble eggs, salt pork, potatoes, fresh milk, and homemade rye bread for breakfast. They would work it off in a morning milking cows, working in the orchard and garden, shoveling out the barn, bringing in the hay, or lifting a transmission out of an automobile or truck. An Italian farmer could easily down a lunch pizza, a draught of homemade wine, and some fruit and feel fully equipped and energized for an afternoon in the vineyard or olive grove. Years ago, members of the Pima tribe (of modern-day Arizona and Mexico) had no weight problems; they scratched and hoed the earth all day to grow corn and beans. Today, with little work to be had on reservations and easy availability of processed foods, their descendants are prone to obesity and diabetes.

Such is the yin and yang of our food. It can be a blessing or a poison, depending on how we manage it.

A BALANCING ACT

A fit life is a result of a multitude of factors. Many people focus almost exclusively on their weight as a life and health problem. Though being overweight is certainly a risk, there is more to it than that. When patients come to see me and ask advice about losing pounds, I first ask them about their exercise pattern. This almost invariably engenders a downcast face, a hopeless shrug of the shoulders, and an upward gesture of the hands imploring my understanding.

Some rules of thumb are essential to the person attempting nonsurgical weight loss. First is the fact that the fundamental determinant of body weight is energy balance: energy in versus energy out. Energy in is composed of all foods consumed in the form of proteins, lipids, and carbohydrates. Energy out includes that required for basal metabolism (accounting for approximately 75 percent of total energy expenditure), *thermogenesis* (the body creating heat, which accounts for approximately 10 percent), and physical activity (accounting for approximately 15 to 30 percent). A net negative 3,500 calories over the course of, say, two weeks will lead to approximately one pound of weight loss. Sustain for three months, and a person can lose over ten pounds.

A second valuable rule of thumb is that a 200-pound person walking at three miles per hour (slow to moderate pace) will burn approximately three calories per minute, or ninety calories during a thirty-minute walk. Avoidance of a single 140-calorie twelve-ounce soft drink is equivalent to walking for approximately forty-five minutes. Do the numbers!

Eating Mindfully

Here is an exercise I learned from my friend and colleague, Jon Kabat-Zinn, who teaches mindfulness-based stress reduction. *Mindfulness* is moment-to-moment, intentional, nonjudgmental awareness and allows us to experience each moment of our lives more deeply, compassionately, and peacefully. When it comes to eating, part of our fast-food-society mindset is nonmindful eating. Hurry up—eat standing in front of the television or computer—grab a drive-through meal—gobble while driving—and move on to the next task of the day.

This exercise in *mindful eating* can affect your eating behavior, help you better control your weight, improve your digestion, and set the stage for better digestive wellness.

RAISIN' YOUR FOOD CONSCIOUSNESS: AN ADVENTURE IN MINDFUL EATING

This exercise, adapted from Kabat-Zinn (1990), demonstrates how enjoyment of your food starts in the brain, not in the mouth. Eating and drinking more deliberately, more mindfully, can help reduce overconsumption, obesity, indigestion, gas, heartburn, dyspepsia, and more. Try this exercise and apply some of the principles to the next three meals you eat to make them more mindful.

1. Start with a bowl of raisins.

2. Reach toward them as you normally would.

3. But pick just one raisin.

4. Don't put it in your mouth right away, but look at it carefully.

5. Notice the folds, the color, the little belly button where the stem was attached to the grape.

6. Next, hold it next to your ear and rub it. Notice the soft sounds it makes.

7. Bring it to your nose and detect the sweet, fruity aroma.

8. Rub it gently on your lips, noticing the soft roughness.

9. This should all take a couple of minutes at the least.

10. Then, put it into your mouth, but don't bite or chew it. Move it around with your tongue, feeling its texture. Move it from one side of your mouth to the other. Is the saliva starting to flow? Don't bite it yet!

11. Next, gently close your teeth on it without chewing. Notice the burst of flavor flowing into the saliva throughout your mouth.

12. Finally, chew slowly, deliberately, enjoying each bite as a burst of flavor and enjoyment.

Compare this to the last time you ate raisins by grabbing a bunch at a time and putting them into your mouth in gobs. Which experience was more enjoyable?

Try slowing down your next three meals—enjoy! Next try it at least for one meal daily for three days, then three weeks. Soon, you'll be in a positive habit of mindfulness-based eating. This approach improves digestion, will likely lower your calorie intake, and helps to make food a joy rather than a bad habit.

For the first few days you try this, make some notes in a journal or on your computer about how this kind of eating feels. How is it different from how you usually eat? What kind of pleasure did you get from eating that you don't ordinarily get? Are you more aware of what you put in your mouth and whether it is healthy for you or not? Do you notice any changes in your digestion, fullness, elimination? Do you notice any changes in your stress level?

Getting Exercise

If you haven't exercised in a while, you are in company with about 60 percent of Americans who don't exercise regularly. In order to avoid injury or overstress your heart, joints, muscles, and other organs, you shouldn't try to go from zero to sixty in a two-week period. For those over forty, checking with your doctor or even getting a stress test is recommended before starting any vigorous exercise program. That being said, the benefits of exercise to your digestive health and overall wellness are so great that you should get a physical exam before you decide *not* to exercise. A healthy adult lifestyle ought to include a total of thirty to sixty minutes of exercise daily.

EXERCISE LOG

Describe your weekly exercise program. Start with the type of exercise, and then list how often you do each one.

How many times a week do you do the following and for how long?

Aerobics (active movement, like walking, swimming, running, calisthenics, or sports)

Resistance (muscle-building exercises, like weight training or isometrics)

_____

Flexibility (stretching, like yoga or tai chi)

_____

Balance (sports requiring good hand-eye coordination, like tennis, or yoga, tai chi, step exercises, or Wii Fit)

_____

Recording your exercise program is a way to be accountable to yourself. Current Centers for Disease Control (2008) guidelines recommend a minimum of 150 minutes a week of some type of aerobic exercise, plus two sessions of muscle-strengthening activities. You can do a moderate-intensity aerobic activity, such as brisk walking, in as little as ten-minute segments and add up the minutes to achieve the desired total.

Keeping a Food Diary

Keeping a food diary can help you begin to take charge of your diet. Simply writing down what you eat and how much you consume can start you on the path toward a more healthful diet.

ONE-DAY FOOD DIARY

Keep a diary of everything you eat today. How many times did you eat?

Describe your breakfast:

_____

_____

Describe your lunch:

_____

_____

Describe your dinner:

_____

_____

List other calories such as snacks and drinks, including after-dinner snacks, alcohol, soft drinks, etc.

_____

_____

What did you notice about your eating habits?

_____

_____

THE FOURTEEN-DAY FOOD DIARY

Using the following worksheet, write down everything you eat for breakfast, lunch, and dinner, plus any snacks, for two consecutive weeks.

Also describe your exercise program within this two-week diary. It is best to do this using the FITT model (frequency, intensity, type, and time). For the first week, just record what kind of exercise you did and for how long and how hard you did it. For week two, use the FITT model to get you in the habit of thinking of your exercise systematically.

It will be interesting to compare what you record with what you recorded in the previous exercise log and one-day food diary. Most overweight people who complete a fourteen-day diet diary will start to lose weight, even without consciously changing their eating habits. There is something about recording and observing your intake that starts to break automatic habitual patterns.

If you are like most people I have known, doing this exercise will be an "aha!" experience. There is an element of surprise and reality shock. Change starts with awareness.

FOURTEEN-DAY FOOD DIARY

	Day 1	Day 2	Day 3	Day 4	Day 5	Day 6	Day 7
Breakfast							
Lunch							
Dinner							
Snacks							
Exercise: Include type of exercise, how hard (easy, moderate, heavy), and duration							

	Day 8	Day 9	Day 10	Day 11	Day 12	Day 13	Day 14
Breakfast							
Lunch							
Dinner							
Snacks							
Exercise: Include type of exercise, how hard (easy, moderate, heavy), and duration							

EATING WELL FOR GOOD HEALTH

The previous exercises in this chapter have made you more aware of your eating and exercise habits and what you'd like to change. The remaining exercises in this chapter will help you develop a better diet for good gut and overall health.

BACK-TO-THE-FUTURE EXERCISE

Look at your fourteen-day food diary again and write down the things you would like to change. For example, "I would change my daily intake of fiber and omega-3 rich foods by adding the following foods." Or "I would add some tai chi or yoga three times weekly to my resistance and aerobic exercises, and plan to start by taking a class at the local gym."

You can do this now if you'd like, though much of the information in the chapters ahead will help you develop a more comprehensive wellness plan to round out your goals and activities. Plan to come back at the end of the book to redo this exercise.

Once you have written down what you would like to change, put this memo in an envelope with your address and have a friend mail it to you in three to six months. Or paste it into your electronic calendar, so it pops up daily for a week or so in three to six months.

Change takes time. Reminders like this help keep you tuned in to what you have already decided is good for your long-term physical and digestive wellness. This exercise will help remind you in the future of what you planned to do today. It also will help keep you accountable to yourself (and no one else) on how well you are doing with your overall wellness program.

Wellness Inventory

Since behavioral change can be so difficult, revisiting your goals regularly is a great way to stay on track. You might want to sign up for an online program like the Wellness Inventory (see the resources at the back of the book). This assessment program covers all areas of health, from food and exercise to stress, spirituality, social connections, and more. You fill out a questionnaire on your overall lifestyle habits and decide which ones you are willing to change now. You then select three to five items to work on and indicate how often you want to be reminded of your goals. An electronic reminder system like this can be a bit annoying at first until you realize you are sending it to yourself to stay on track with your new nutrition, fitness, and overall wellness plan.

Here is a short quiz you can take to get a closer look at your current diet.

HOW HEALTHY IS YOUR DIET?

After careful thought, circle your answers to the following questions, and then add up your points (the numbers in parentheses) to find your total score.

1. How many servings of fruit do you normally eat each day (one-half cup fresh or dried fruit, one medium piece of fruit, or one cup unsweetened juice)?

    A. None (-2)

    B. One (0)

    C. Two to three (+2)

    D. Four or more (+3)

2. How many vegetable servings do you normally eat each day (one cup leafy greens or one-half cup any other veggie, raw or cooked)?

    A. None (-4)

    B. One (0)

    C. Two (+1)

    D. Three (+2)

    E. Four or more (+3)

3. How many different varieties of vegetables do you eat in a normal month?

    A. Two or less (-4)

    B. Three to four (0)

    C. Five to six (+1)

    D. Seven to eight (+3)

    E. Nine or more (+4)

4. How many times do you eat dried beans or peas (legumes, lentils, chickpeas, kidney beans, green peas, etc.) in a normal week?

    A. Never (-2)

    B. One to two (0)

    C. Three to four (+1)

D. Five to six (+2)

E. Seven or more (+3)

5. How many times do you eat red meat in a normal week?

    A. Six or more (-4)

    B. Four to five (-3)

    C. One to three (-1)

    D. Less than once a week (+2)

    E. Never (+3)

6. How many times do you eat in a fast-food restaurant in a normal week?

    A. Six or more (-5)

    B. Four to five (-4)

    C. One to three (-3)

    D. Less than once a week (-2)

    E. Never (0)

7. In a typical day, what do you drink most often?

    A. Soda (regular or diet) (-4)

    B. Decaffeinated coffee or tea (0)

    C. Milk or fruit juice (0)

    D. Caffeinated coffee or tea (+1)

    E. Herbal tea, green tea, or water (+3)

8. How many twelve-ounce cans of soda do you drink in a normal day?

    A. Six or more (-5)

    B. Four to five (-4)

    C. Two to three (-3)

    D. One (-2)

    E. Less than one (-1)

    F. None (0)

9. How often do you eat fish in a typical week?

    A. Never (-2)

    B. Once (+1)

    C. Twice (+2)

    D. Three to five times (+3)

10. In a typical week, how often do you eat whole grains (100 percent whole-grain bread, whole oats, brown rice, quinoa, whole rye crackers)?

    A. Never (-3)

    B. One to two times a week (-1)

    C. Three to four times a week (0)

    D. Five to six times a week (+1)

    E. One or more times a day (+3)

11. How often do you eat sweets such as cookies, cakes, or ice cream?

    A. One or more times a day (-3)

    B. Every other day (-2)

    C. Twice a week (-1)

    D. Once a week (0)

    E. Two to three times a month (+1)

    F. Rarely (+3)

Your total score: _____

Scoring:

22 to 28 = Great eating habits

17 to 21 = Pretty good eating habits

10 to 16 = Needs some improvement

9 or less = Needs much improvement; try to change one habit at a time.

Survey adapted from the Institute for Functional Medicine

How did you do? Could your diet use some improvement? The next section will help you make some positive changes.

Pyramid Schemes

Food is good and needs to be balanced with exercise. But what kind of food and how much, and how should we prepare it? Healthy food pyramids, designed for practically every taste and ethnic preference, emphasize plant-based, low-fat options as a base, with lower levels of carbohydrates, protein, fats, and sugars as you move up the pyramid. You want to strive for a diet of whole foods with minimal processing, lots of fruits and vegetables, whole grains, low fat or healthy fat, and protein sources such as salmon, skinless turkey breast, lean meats, beans, and nuts. This holds true across a spectrum of food pyramids, though the types and proportions of foods vary.

Many attempts have been made to help distribute caloric intake across a variety of food groups. Interestingly, children, when offered a variety of foods, may not seem to be eating a balanced diet over a few days or so, but they generally take in all their bodies need over a longer period. So don't be hung up on eating perfectly every day or per meal, but instead try to move to a healthier diet on average over a period of a couple weeks or a month. That is why the fourteen-day food diary is really more useful than a single-day snapshot in helping you plan a digestive wellness diet.

Each meal counts. Each food choice is potentially health-promoting or disease-causing. A salad-and-juice fast with a colon or liver cleanse for a few days doesn't mean you ought to be slobbering down sliders, cheeseburgers, soda, pizza, and tacos daily for the rest of the month. "Everything in moderation, even moderation" is my motto. Or as another author said, "Eat food. Not too much. Mostly plants" (Pollan 2008). Food pyramids summarize the best medical and nutritional science, conveniently illustrating optimal proportions, portions, mixes, numbers of servings, and types of foods. Healthy food pyramids for Mediterranean, Asian, Latin American, soul food, vegetarian, vegan, and other dietary choices are available online (see resources for more information).

FOOD PYRAMID OPTIONS

1. Choose a food pyramid and attach a copy to the front of your refrigerator. Keep another copy visible where you normally jot down your shopping list. Use it.

2. Develop a healthy menu plan for a week, using the pyramid guidelines. Consult your favorite cookbook. Go shopping. Start cooking. Finish by eating!

Social Influences

Family and friends can be a major influence on your food choices. Suppose that your friends invite you to lunch at a certain Mexican restaurant. Perhaps this restaurant offers little in the way of healthy food. What do you do to stay sociable and avoid either being a hermit or getting unhealthy? Doing so requires a bit of courage, humility, and, to make it work, firmness in your choices. Arriving at the restaurant where everyone is eating heaping platters of cheese-covered nachos, fat-fried chimichangas, and heavily caloried burritos, take your seat and quietly order a chicken taco salad and an iced tea or some grilled fish a la casa. Watch as your friends surreptitiously review their menu choices and perhaps move from burrito to cabrito, from beef to fish taco, or from fatty to more fruit- and vegetable-laden courses.

Family meals can be challenging. Glorious food changes in families occur slowly. What you bring home in the shopping cart offers the kids some positive or unhealthy options. Is it carrots and celery sticks for snacks, or crackers and cheese, or jujubes? At large family gatherings, you can increase the number of healthier foods by bringing more salads and vegetables. Bring a special healthy covered dish and make sure it is delicious. Or just eat less of what is offered without being impolite. Above all, avoid judgmental comments that will make others uncomfortable. Lead by example.

IMPROVING YOUR DIETARY PATTERNS

Make a list below of the kinds of foods your family and friends eat regularly that you know are less than optimally healthy:

_____

_____

_____

_____

Now describe the kinds of foods that would still be culturally appropriate with your family and friends but that you know are healthier:

_____

_____

_____

_____

_____

_____

Here is where the rubber meets the road. Describe the kinds of behaviors you could implement to change your dietary patterns in your social setting. Examples: "Bring my own healthy lunch and eat it in the lunchroom; offer to cook a turkey breast or salmon fillet and grilled veggies instead of steaks and ribs at the family BBQ; suggest multiple types of salads at family and social events instead of larger entrées."

_____

_____

_____

_____

_____

CONCLUSION

It is important to make healthful food choices as well as to enjoy the full range of social and cultural aspects surrounding food. Making small changes in your food and exercise choices is clearly the best way to prevent many chronic diseases, such as obesity, diabetes, hypertension, and heart disease. Your gut can only make the best of what you choose to feed it. As the saying goes, "Garbage in, garbage out." By working through the simple exercises in this chapter, you and your family can start on a healthier approach to "glorious food" and begin to radiate good health.

Chapter 3

Eating Bugs and Other Gastrointestinal Delights

The Benefits of Probiotics

Eating bugs may seem an unappetizing prospect, but this chapter shows that regularly eating the bacteria in fermented foods like yogurt can substantially improve your health.

Bacteria in your gut are essential to digestion and elimination functions and key to your immunity and your body's health. Probiotics, single or mixed cultures of live microbes, can have beneficial effects on health by altering the gastrointestinal microbiota (intestinal bacteria). Probiotics are present in many common and traditional foods.

Start with breakfast. There are many possible ways to get your metabolism and digestion going for the day, and eating a good breakfast is a great way to start your day in a healthy direction. People who eat breakfast live longer, have an easier time with weight problems, and give their attitude a boost (Guralnik and Kaplan 1989). Furthermore, eating bugs for breakfast regularly introduces healthy bacteria (probiotics) into your system.

Breakfasts that contain whole grains, healthy fats, and high fiber offer a slower, healthier absorption curve than those that don't. Such foods cause less rapid fluctuations in insulin and blood sugar. They help keep you full and happy until your next meal. Such healthy breakfast foods as yogurt and kefir contain health-promoting bugs. Other great breakfast options include salmon, soymilk, hummus, organic peanut butter, and high omega-3 eggs. Always consider including whole-grain cereals like granola and oatmeal and whole-grain breads like various kinds of Ezekiel bread (sprouted grains, sesame) containing at least three grams of fiber per slice.

BUGS CAN BE GOOD FOR YOUR HEALTH

You may not realize that one of the largest organs in your body is made up almost entirely of bacteria. Over 400 different microbial species live in your gut, with thirty to forty species making up 99 percent of the total. The estimated weight of this *biomass* of bugs is around six pounds. These microorganisms live as single cells or in colonies called *biofilms,* highly ordered and made up of multiple species. They cooperate with each other and prevent other bacteria and viruses that cause infections. Probiotics contribute to the formation of health-promoting biofilms and thus contribute to the inhibition of invasive bacteria and the formation of unhealthy bacterial biofilms.

In other words, bugs are good for you, at least certain kinds are. I know most of us think of bacteria as bad actors, causing diseases like strep throat, pneumonia, meningitis, and tuberculosis. That is true, but probiotics are a different breed of bug, so to speak, and actually protect against certain diseases.

A newborn's gut is sterile and does not contain significant numbers of bacteria. So how do all those bugs get in there?

The truth is that bacteria are everywhere and are an essential part of the ecology of the planet. They live in soil, water, the ocean, and air, and, of course, they live in and on animals, humans, plants, and even rocks. There is no escaping bacteria. Whether you were born by normal vaginal delivery or cesarean section, whether you were breast-fed or bottle-fed, as a baby you were inoculated with certain organisms from your mother and the environment. These grow and multiply within the gut over time.

Babies who arrive by vaginal birth and are breast-fed have a healthier mix of bugs in their gut than C-section and bottle-fed babies (Kligler and Cohrssen 2008). Solid research (the "hygiene hypothesis") shows that kids must be exposed to a certain amount of "dirt," including the bacteria associated with it, to have healthy lives. Those with little exposure to natural environmental bacteria and other *antigens* (factors that activate the immune system) may experience higher levels of allergies, asthma, eczema, and other immune-related diseases later in life (Litonjua et al. 2002). Mothers who take probiotics prior to delivery can, in high-risk allergenic families, reduce risk of eczema in their offspring (Kalliomaki et al. 2003; Kalliomaki et al. 2007).

Shopping for Probiotics

So, what foods should you add to your shopping list? The following foods are jam-packed with probiotics:

- yogurt

- kefir

- sauerkraut

- milk

- buttermilk

- kimchi

- some cheeses (aged cheeses, probiotic-enhanced cheeses, cottage cheese)

- miso

- tempeh

- kombucha mushroom

Yogurt is probably the best-known probiotic-enriched food and is a healthful part of breakfast, whether over cereal, with fruit or granola, by itself, or as part of a smoothie. Kefir is another probiotic delight for breakfast. Kefir is a liquid dairy product, somewhere in consistency between buttermilk and yogurt. It pours rather than being spooned and is delicious over whole-grain cereal. It can substitute for a smoothie.

When shopping for probiotics, look for a statement about "live" or "active" cultures on these products. Manufacturers are increasingly realizing the health benefits (and marketing value) of probiotics for their product lines.

Probiotics are also available in capsules or tablets. Refrigerated varieties in your health-food store are likely to be the most potent and active.

EXERCISE: ADDING BUGS TO YOUR DIET

List some ways you can add probiotics into your diet next week. Bugs for breakfast is an easy place to start. For example, "On Monday morning, I'll have cereal with …" or "On Saturday, I'll drink some kefir with my toast," or "I'll get a supplement." Make it specific, listing when, what, and perhaps where:

_____

_____

_____

_____

_____

_____

_____

Since the effects of probiotics generally take some time, you may not notice an immediate effect on your health. The important thing is to trust the wisdom of your body and its delicate ability to adjust the microbiotic environment with regularly ingested probiotics. Listen to your body as you ingest probiotics to know when enough is enough (when your post-antibiotic diarrhea resolves, if you are taking probiotics for this problem) or if you've had too much (you experience a lot of flatulence or bloating).

Continue taking probiotics for your long-term health, and change the kind of probiotics every few months, just to give your digestive system some variety of species, particularly if you are taking capsule formulations, in which these are usually detailed.

While current research supports the benefits of probiotics for a variety of gastrointestinal conditions, the exact species, dose, and duration of intake remain uncertain for some conditions.

Common Probiotic Bacteria

The most common bacteria found in probiotic foods and supplements are the following:

- _Lactobacillus GG_

- _Lactobacillus casei_

- _Lactobacillus acidophilus_

- _Lactobacillus planatarum_

- _Lactobacillus reuteri_

- _Bifidobacterium bifidum/longum_

- *Saccharomyces boulardii*

- *Streptococcus thermophilus*

Numerous studies demonstrate probiotics' specific functions in the gut, of promoting resistance to colonization of unhealthy bacteria and producing antibacterial substances (Bengmark 1998). Probiotics increase production of mucus, preventing bacterial attachment. Some evidence suggests they help neutralize dietary carcinogens and modulate the activity of inflammatory chemicals in the system (Rolfe 2000).

Probiotics compete with other gut bacteria for nutrients and inhibit bacterial adhesion at sites on the intestinal membranes. Through these activities, probiotics significantly enhance immune system defenses.

Prebiotics Are Good Too

Probiotics feed on *prebiotics*, or nondigestible nutrients. We all need nourishment, right? Prebiotics are colon food for probiotics; they provide a substrate for healthy bacteria to grow in your gut.

Prebiotics selectively stimulate activity of one or more colonic microorganisms that promote health and well-being of the host. These *oligosaccharides* come from foods like onions, asparagus, chicory, bananas, and artichokes. By adding prebiotic foods to your diet or adding supplement capsules to the probiotics that you consume, you can maximize their effects.

HEALTH BENEFITS OF PROBIOTICS

Probiotics research indicates reduction in the time course of infectious or antibiotic-induced diarrhea (Allen et al. 2004; Vanderhoof 2000), reduction in the risk of skin allergy (atopic eczema) in infants and children when their mothers take probiotics prenatally (Kalliomaki et al. 2007), and reduction in symptoms of irritable bowel syndrome (Brenner et al. 2009).

Individuals vary in their needs for probiotics, and the large variety of types of probiotics and probiotic mixtures makes it challenging to sort out the full range of data. Probiotics may be useful in many conditions of the gastrointestinal system:

- *dysbiosis* (imbalance between healthy and unhealthy intestinal bacteria)

- gut infections such as *Helicobacter pylori* (*H. pylori*), traveler's diarrhea, AIDS-related diarrhea, and pediatric/infantile diarrhea

- lactose intolerance

- inflammatory bowel disease

- leaky gut

- colic

- cystic fibrosis

- liver disease

Probiotics may also improve the immune system and help with the following related conditions:

- inflammatory disorders of the gut, the joints, and other organ systems

- recurrent sinus and respiratory infections

- vaginal yeast infections, especially after antibiotic use

- allergic rhinitis

- atopy

- asthma

- immuno-augmentation of vaccines: boosting response to effect of vaccination

- genitourinary infection

The Case of Ruth's Diarrhea

Ruth is a patient of mine. A sixty-two-year-old white woman with a chronic lung disease, she had been treated three months previously with antibiotics and steroids for her worsening condition. She developed a gut infection, which led to profuse, watery diarrhea twelve to fifteen times a day, and she was treated with yet another antibiotic because of a secondary infection in her colon. Despite this standard therapy, the diarrhea persisted and Ruth was admitted to the hospital with dehydration requiring IV fluids. During a ten-day hospital stay, an extensive gastrointestinal workup was done to rule out common and rare causes of chronic diarrhea. Her white blood cell count was elevated, suggesting inflammation or infection, so another antibiotic was given. Despite the high white count, her blood, stool, and urine cultures did not show any bacteria.

I saw Ruth on weekend hospital rounds and suspected that an imbalance of healthy and unhealthy bacteria in her gut (dysbiosis)was the underlying cause of her persistent and intractable diarrhea. I stopped all antibiotics and placed her on high-dose Lactobacillus capsules daily. Within two days, the diarrhea had resolved, and we stopped IV fluids and she returned home.

This case illustrates that medical treatments can sometimes cause problems that need probiotics for recovery. Medicines like antibiotics, steroids, antacids, and others can affect gut health, creating problems related to an abnormal overgrowth of bacteria in the gut (see chapter 10 for more details). Like a weed taking over your garden, these problems of overgrowth of bacteria and other kinds of gut infections and chronic diarrhea can be improved through the use of probiotics. In Ruth's case, probiotics helped restore intestinal bacterial balance, solving her serious problems.

How to Take Probiotic Supplements

How you prefer to take probiotic supplements depends on you and why you're taking them. Here are some general principles:

- Take on an empty stomach—may take as a single dose or divided before meals.

- Space three to four hours after taking an antibiotic and continue for at least two weeks after completing treatment.

- Take at least 1 billion organisms per dose for health maintenance.

- Typical daily doses should be in the range of 3 to 10 billion units and may be continued indefinitely.

- After taking antibiotics and for certain conditions, you may take 20 to 30 billion units a day or more, the length of time depending on your response and on the condition.

The length of intake of probiotics is uncertain for many conditions, and the science continues to evolve regarding what species, strain, or mix of species is optimal for certain conditions. This ought not to dissuade you from taking bugs for breakfast or anytime. Even non-viable organisms may have benefits by blocking bacterial adherence to the gut wall. If you don't have the fortified or live cultures, you may still experience a health benefit. I recommend that you refrigerate most products to ensure the maximum survival of bacteria.

SIDE EFFECTS

Some people experience bloating, flatulence, and mild abdominal discomfort. Probiotics are safe at even extremely high doses in the range of 400 to 500 billion units. There is a rare risk of *bacteremia* (germs in the bloodstream) in immuno-compromised or severely ill people or in children with a condition known as *short gut syndrome* (Young and Vanderhoof 2004). Infections have never been seen with *Bifidobacterium*, though some infections in severely ill patients have been seen with *Lactobacillus* (Salminen et al. 2002).

Premature infants may also be at higher risk, though some neonatologists have treated them with probiotics and found reduction in a serious condition called *necrotizing enterocolitis* (Ruemmele et al. 2009). There are no known interactions of probiotic supplements with medications or other supplements.

CONCLUSION

Probiotics ought to be part of your healthy diet throughout the day, added easily through the many foods listed here as well as probiotic supplements. They help protect your system against illnesses and help treat some established conditions. Adding this food or supplement source to your diet can safely and cheaply reap enormous health benefits.

Chapter 4

The SuperFoods

The Best Researched
Foods for Gut Health
and Overall Wellness

When you eat, you're giving your body raw materials for living. What you consume affects all aspects of your body's functioning. Your food choices affect health not only in the digestive system but in every body system. The body is like a factory where raw materials are processed. High-quality materials are processed into high-quality products. Eating well helps build healthy bones, blood, heart, muscles, eyes, kidneys, brain, and other essential components.

The wonderful thing is that you do have a choice! What you decide to eat becomes part of your body, your mind, and perhaps your spiritual path.

So, what foods should you eat regularly, and how much of these should you eat? Chapter 2 discussed how food pyramids recommend food types, proportions, and frequencies. This chapter will make more specific recommendations, inspired by the work of a wonderful physician named Steve Pratt and his SuperFoodsRx series of books (Pratt and Kolberg 2009; Brazilian and Pratt; Pratt and Matthews 2005; Pratt 2004). Dr. Pratt is an ophthalmologist, specializing in eye disease. He extended his research and writing into nutrition after seeing a family member suffering from near blindness due to macular degeneration, a condition that leads to functional blindness in many elderly. When he noticed that some patients after eye surgery seemed to have more efficient wound healing, he wondered if nutrition was the key.

MEET THE SUPERFOODS

Dr. Pratt identified fourteen foods that offer extraordinary properties associated with the greatest health benefits, and he popularized the term *SuperFoods* to describe them. Each of these foods has what he calls *sidekicks*, related foods with similar or identical health benefits, and these sidekicks are listed below with each of the primary SuperFoods. The following list of SuperFoods was based on extensive scientific nutritional research and has been confirmed in peer-reviewed studies.

The mission of this chapter is to make these foods a central part of your diet to improve your digestion, skin, eyes, heart, brain, and overall health.

The Original SuperFoods

BEANS

Sidekicks: pinto, navy, great northern, lima, garbanzo (chickpeas), lentils, green beans, sugar snap peas, black beans, and green peas.

As we have become wealthier in our society, our sources of protein include less legumes and more meat. Pity the lowly bean when faced with such competitors as steak, burgers, and pork chops. Yet beans are one of the most healthful foods, providing high-quality, low-fat protein with B vitamins, iron, potassium, magnesium, and more. Because of their high fiber content, beans help control blood sugar and diabetes, as well as gut problems like diverticulosis, constipation, and hemorrhoids. Their pigments help protect your skin from sun damage. Beans help reduce cardiac risks, cholesterol levels, and possibly cancers of the colon, breast, and prostate. If you get gas from beans, increase the amount you take gradually, soak beans overnight or pressure-cook them, or consider adding a product called Beano to your beans. Chew them slowly to aid in maximum digestion. Aim to eat at least four cup servings per week for maximum benefit (Anderson and

Gustafson 1988; Brown et al. 1999; Graf and Eaton 1993; Kushi, Meyer, and Jacobs 1999; Slattery et al. 1997; Commenges et al. 2000).

BLUEBERRIES

Sidekicks: purple grapes, cranberries, boysenberries, raspberries, strawberries, currants, blackberries, cherries, and all other varieties of fresh, frozen, or dried berries.

This berry group provides a large number of phytochemicals, antioxidants, and nutrients such as polyphenols that protect your eyes, brain, and circulatory system. The fiber content and pectin in berries have traditionally been used for digestive health, particularly for conditions like diarrhea and constipation (Cao et al. 1998; Commenges et al. 2000). Most folks know the benefits of cranberries for urinary tract infections. I like to use berries thoughout the day: in a smoothie, over cereal, or with yogurt for breakfast; as a snack; or for dessert, as an alternative to the sugary desserts offered at restaurants. It is easy to keep frozen berries in the freezer along with the fresh ones, which seem to be in season or available most of the year. Aim for a cup or two daily.

BROCCOLI

Sidekicks: brussels sprouts, cabbage, kale, turnips, cauliflower, collards, bok choy, mustard greens, and Swiss chard.

Among the most super of the SuperFoods, the broccoli group includes such nutrients as iron and calcium, vitamins C, K, and folic acid, carotenoids, and high fiber. They activate detoxification processes in the liver, helping to eliminate unwanted toxins from food and the environment, such as pesticides, herbicides, and other chemicals. The sulfur-containing compounds act as detoxicants, providing anticancer effects for the GI system for colon, stomach, rectal, and lung cancer (Cohen, Kristal, and Stanford 2000; van Poppel et al. 1999). These nutrients also support bone, eye, and heart health. I like to roll thin spears of broccolini in olive oil, add some organic seasoning, and then grill them. Delicious! Broccoli sprouts, extremely high in antioxidants and cancer-fighting power, are great on salads or sandwiches (Nestle 1998). Try to get up to one cup of cooked or raw broccoli or sidekicks into your diet daily.

OATS

Sidekicks: wheat germ, ground flaxseed, brown rice, barley, wheat, buckwheat, rye, millet, bulgur wheat, amaranth, quinoa, triticale, kamut, yellow corn, wild rice, spelt, and couscous.

Whole grains are one of the most healthful foods. Unless you have a sensitivity to gluten or other digestive problem, as discussed in later chapters, they are one of your best sources of protein, fiber, and minerals such as magnesium, potassium, and zinc, and B vitamins. The first food-specific health claim approved by the FDA was for oatmeal: that eating oats reduces cholesterol. The benefits of whole grains go much further. The high fiber helps reduce risk of GI conditions such as diverticulosis and hemorrhoids, helps alleviate irritable bowel syndrome, and also helps stabilize blood sugar and reduce risk of heart disease (Cleveland et al. 2000; S. Liu et al. 2002). Addition of supplemental sidekicks like wheat germ and flaxseed can improve all these conditions further. Whole grains are easy to include at breakfast in your cereal or bread and later in the day as brown rice and other nutritious grains. You need to consume at least five to seven servings daily of the whole-grain family.

ORANGES

Sidekicks: lemons, white and pink grapefruit, kumquats, tangerines, and limes.

Besides being important and easily accessible sources of vitamin C and potassium, citrus fruits contain limonene (especially the peel), flavonoids, and polyphenols, all of which are important antioxidant, anti-inflammatory, antimicrobial, and anticancer agents (Crowell 1999; L. Liu et al. 2002). Oranges and sidekicks also have high amounts of fiber, folic acid, and quercetin. All have been found to improve cardiovascular health and improve immunity. Eating a bit of the skin and white pulp increases the benefits, helps your body absorb more benefits of other polyphenols, such as tea, and can decrease inflammation, blood pressure, and cholesterol (Cao, Sofic, and Prior 1996). High-pulp juice has more nutrient value than low-pulp. You ought to get at least one serving a day of oranges or their sidekicks.

PUMPKIN

Sidekicks: carrots, butternut squash, sweet potatoes, and orange bell peppers.

We tend to think of pumpkin as a seasonal holiday vegetable. In fact, it is a fruit, like melon, is very high in alpha and beta carotenes, and is a rich source of vitamins C and E, potassium, and magnesium. These carotenes help the body produce vitamin A as well. Native Americans, who reputedly brought pumpkin to the first Thanksgiving, may have helped save the early settlers' lives by supplying a food high in disease-fighting nutrients. Improved vision, cancer-risk reduction, lowered heart disease risk, and better skin health all have been found with the carotenoids, like those found in pumpkin and its sidekicks (Ascherio et al. 1999; Bowen et al. 1993; Krinsky 1998). Don't smoke and expect carotenoids to help you, however; they may actually raise the risk of lung cancer in smokers (Albanes et al. 1996). Dr. Pratt's *SuperFoods Rx* (see resources) has several excellent pumpkin recipes to help you enjoy this supernutrient-packed food—and not just during the holidays. Enjoy one-half cup or more of this food group daily.

WILD SALMON

Sidekicks: Alaskan halibut, canned albacore tuna, sardines, herring, trout, sea bass, oysters, and clams.

There are many benefits from the omega-3 essential fatty acids in this group of foods. The fats found in these fish provide numerous health benefits through their anti-inflammatory effects. They reduce risk of gut inflammation; heart problems; arthritis; certain eye conditions, such as macular degeneration; cancer; mental health problems; and more. Even one serving weekly can reduce heart attack and stroke risk (Albert et al. 1998; Bhatnagar and Durrington 2003; Kris-Etherton et al. 2002). The omega-3 level is higher in wild salmon than in farmed salmon and other fish. Canned sockeye can be a low-cost healthful addition to your diet when served on a salad or as a salmon burger, as a fishloaf, or on a sandwich. While there are some issues with eating fish because of potential environmental toxins such as mercury, dioxin, and PCBs (polychlorinated biphenyls), smart shopping can help reduce the risk. Smaller fish like sardines, herring, and trout are less likely to have concentrated toxins than bigger fish such as swordfish, king mackerel, shark, and tilefish. Canned light tuna is lower in mercury than albacore. Eat no more than six ounces of albacore a week, to limit mercury intake. Also, minimize raw sushi tuna to a few pieces a month, as it is also high in mercury.

Try for at least two to four servings of fish weekly. Check with your doctor if you are in a special risk group. Pregnant women and children must be even more careful in their selection of fish.

SOY

Sidekicks: tofu, soymilk, soy nuts, edamame, tempeh, and miso.

Of all the SuperFoods, soy is the one most people in the United States seem to have the least experience with eating. In fact, soy is the most complete plant protein and an excellent meat subsititute. It provides such health benefits as detoxification and hormonal protection, and it contains omega-3 fatty acids, potassium, magnesium, selenium, and vitamins E and folic acid. One important feature of soy is that it contains phytoestrogens, which can block the receptors on cells that connect with circulating estrogen. This reduces menopausal symptoms and reduces the risk of hormone-dependent tumors, such as in the breast, the ovaries, the uterus, and even the prostate and is useful in promoting bone health (Messina et al. 1994). Women who have had breast cancer should speak to their doctors before consuming large amounts of soy or soy/isoflavone supplements, though a large study from Shanghai found that breast cancer survivors who ate more soy were less likely to have a recurrence than those who ate less (Xiao et al. 2009). There are many ways to eat soy. You can snack on soy nuts or cooked pods (edamame), enjoy tofu (bean curd) cooked in some delicious sauce, use soymilk over your cereal, add soy protein powder to a smoothie, or chow down on soy-based meat substitutes like burgers or hot dogs, baked or grille In general, avoid supplements and use whole-food soy products for the best benefits. Im your shopping habits by adding at least one soy product from the list above and experi with a new recipe. The usual amount recommended for health benefit is only fiftee soy protein daily.

SPINACH

Sidekicks: kale, collard, Swiss chard, mustard greens, turnip greens, bok choy, romaine lettuce, and orange bell peppers.

Remember Popeye the sailor man in the cartoons? His strength and vitality were attributed to spinach. And without doubt, spinach is a top SuperFood and epitomizes the leafy greens. Either cooked or raw, spinach is a cornucopia of nutritious components, including iron, carotenoids, vitamins B, C, and E, omega-3 fatty acids, mutiple minerals, antioxidants, and polyphenols. These days, spinach is easy to buy prewashed in tidy bags for salads or cooking. It's delicious in salad, in a whole-grain rice-spinach casserole, as a cooked vegetable, in soups, in omelets, or on sandwiches. I even enjoy spinach for breakfast with a slice of whole-grain bread smeared with hummus, with onion, tomato, and smoked salmon. Spinach supports eye health through lutein- and zeaxanthin-containing carotenoids. Useful for protecting you from heart disease and cancer, it may also prevent cognitive decline (Colditz et al. 1985; John et al. 2002; Slattery et al. 2000; Morris et al. 2006). Popeye was not only strong, he was smart! Go for at least one to two cups of spinach or sidekicks daily.

TEA, GREEN OR BLACK

Besides water, tea is the most consumed beverage in the world. Fortunately, research shows that tea has extensive health benefits. While most research has been done on green tea, any form of tea is beneficial. Tea contains polyphenols and a chemical class called *epigallocatechins* that have anticancer effects, improve heart health, and improve dental health (Heilbrun, Nomura, and Stemmermann 1986; Ahmad and Mukhtar 1999; Duffy et al. 2001; Geleijnse et al. 2002; Hegarty, May, and Khaw 2000). If you are trying to avoid caffeine, know that tea is lower in caffeine than coffee. You can decaffeinate your tea easily by brewing a pot and pouring out the liquid, along with the caffeine, then adding back hot water to the same tea bags. When you enjoy tea, squeeze the teabag in order to extract the polyphenols that are so healthy for you. Adding some citrus to tea or adding pepper to a meal when you're drinking tea will help you absorb more of tea's healthful components. To get the most benefit from tea, drink it fresh-brewed or quickly

maker gives me freshly chilled iced tea in a few minutes. A pitcher of green tea

nk to sip and is calorie free. Try to drink at least a cup daily.

higher amounts, even as many as ten cups daily (McKay and

pink grapefruit, Japanese persimmons, red-fleshed papaya, and

If you have never heard of lycopene, it's time you did. Tomatoes are the most common source (along with their sidekicks) of this red pigment–derived chemical. Lycopene has been shown in research to lower the risks of prostate, lung, and stomach cancer (Giovannucci 1999). In addition to lycopene, tomatoes are rich in carotenoids, vitamins C and B, fiber, and some minerals. They are also good for eye health and reduce risk of heart disease (Upritchard, Sutherland, and Mann 2000). One study showed improved mental function in elderly nuns who had high levels of lycopene in their systems (Snowdon, Gross, and Butler 1996). Tomatoes, believe it or not, once thought to be poisonous (Goodwin and Goodwin 1984), have become one of our most popular foods. Canned tomatoes and sauces have even higher concentrations of lycopene, carotenoids, vitamins, and antioxidants, so you can feel good about making pasta sauces, chili, and soups when ripe tomatoes aren't available. Try making pizza a SuperFood by ordering the vegetarian variety on a whole-wheat crust and adding an extra dose of tomato sauce and chicken grilled in olive oil. The kids will enjoy it too, and it's good for you!

SKINLESS TURKEY BREAST

Sidekick: skinless chicken breast.

Like pumpkin, turkey used to be just for the holidays, but you can consume this low-fat, healthy meat year-round, and you don't need to face the daunting task of cooking a whole bird. You can cook turkey breasts and even turkey sausage. Ground turkey breast can be easily used in burgers, meat sauces, or meat loaf, as taco/burrito meat, and in soup, pasta, and more. Turkey is a great source of protein, is low in fat, and contains essential B vitamins and selenium and zinc, making turkey good for the heart and immune system (Clark et al. 1996; Eaton and Konner 1985). Skinless chicken breast has many of the same benefits as turkey. Avoid both the calories and saturated fat of unskinned chicken or turkey breast. Other low-fat meats are buffalo/bison, which is even lower in fat than salmon and offers a dose of delicious red meat. Though not in the turkey SuperFood class à la Dr. Pratt, it has many of the same benefits of turkey with the additional vitamin B_{12} and iron offered by red meat. You can use ground buffalo just as you would use ground turkey breast. At the grocery store, look for the ground turkey breast or other turkey meats in the freezer section (bison for variety) and substitute them for ground beef or red meat. Though the U.S. diet is not likely to be low in protein, try to use skinless turkey breast or skinless chicken breast three to four times a week as a substitute for other meat proteins.

WALNUTS

Sidekicks: Almonds, pistachios, sesame seeds, peanuts, pumpkin and sunflower seeds, macadamia nuts, pecans, hazelnuts, and cashews.

Nuts, a great source of omega-3 fatty acids, have numerous health benefits. They are an excellent source of fiber, vitamins, protein, and minerals. They are also high in calories, so consuming a handful per day is adequate without increasing your risk of gaining weight. The good news is that eating nuts can reduce your risks of developing heart disease, diabetes, and certain kinds of cancer, such as colorectal, endometrial, prostate, oral, and breast (Albert et al. 2002; Jiang et al. 2002; Lovejoy et al. 2002; Kris-Etherton, Harris, and Appel 2003; Jenab et al. 2004). Pumpkin and sunflower seeds are members of the nut group. Remember the joy of peanut butter in your childhood? It is still a great way to get nuts into your diet. I prefer Laura Scudder's brand of natural peanut butter without trans fat. Slather it on some whole-grain bread at breakfast or at lunch. Nuts and seeds will be beneficial to your health at about an ounce or so a day.

YOGURT

Sidekick: kefir (a fermented dairy product like yogurt but more liquid).

You've heard of yogurt, yes? How about kefir? Kefir is a dairy product that tastes like yogurt but is more liquid and pourable. In chapter 3, you learned about the benefits of fermented products like yogurt on your gut health. You can easily add kefir or yogurt to your breakfast, sprinkling granola over yogurt, eating yogurt with fruit, or pouring kefir on your cereal. If you're in a rush, you can chug kefir on the way to work. Make yogurt or kefir a low-fat form of protein in your diet at the dose of one to two cups daily.

Additional SuperFoods and Sidekicks

These additional SuperFoods and their sidekicks will make your eating choices even more varied, enjoyable, and healthy. Include these in your diet plan for snacks and as part of your meals, and you'll feel better in the short term and in the long run.

Apples. Sidekick: pears. High in antioxidants, anti-inflammatory, high fiber. Eat the skin.

Avocado. Sidekicks: asparagus, artichokes. Healthy fats, prebiotic, anti-inflammatory, rich in potassium, magnesium, vitamin E, folic acid.

Dark chocolate. Yumm. Get over 70 percent cocoa content for the most natural antioxidant power and polyphenols. Limit to 100 calories a day!

Dried SuperFruits. These include raisins, dates, prunes, figs, apricots, blueberries, cranberries, cherries, currants. Great snacks with lots of fiber, potassium, polyphenols, and other phytonutrients. Add to cereal, desserts, yogurt, or eat alone. Go organic when possible.

Extra virgin olive oil. Sidekick: canola oil. The healthful cooking, marinating, and dressing oils of choice, rich in healthy monounsaturated omega-9 fatty acids, vitamin E, polyphenols, plant sterols, and carotenoids.

Honey. Healthy sweetness, rich in prebiotics, antioxidants. Rich tradition of healing for skin, GI tract, and respiratory disease, as one of the oldest healing substances known to man.

Kiwi. Sidekicks: pineapple, guava. Rich in antioxidant vitamins, such as C and E, anti-inflammatory substances, polyphenols, carotenoids.

Onions. Sidekicks: garlic, scallions, shallots, leeks, chives. Sulfur-containing quercetin, vitamins, and minerals like selenium that are anti-inflammatory, antibiotic, detoxifying, and immune boosting. Excellent prebiotic source.

Pomegranates. Sidekick: plums. Powerful antioxidant and other possible health benefits ranging from lowering blood pressure to improving hearing and eye function. Easiest to consume as juice, though seeds can be blended into a smoothie.

SuperSpices

Everyone uses spices in cooking, but you may not realize that in addition to improving the flavor of foods, they contain extensive health benefits. All traditions and cultures have long used spices as preservatives and for their medicinal qualities, and they can add that extra something to a meal and to your health. Rosemary, a favorite of mine, was traditionally used to preserve lamb and other meats due to its plant oils with antibiotic properties. Now, we commonly think of rosemary as essential to a good leg of lamb, not knowing it was once a preservative before there was refrigeration. Such preservatives as this might help preserve you! The following spices may provide these helpful properties:

- cinnamon: lowering blood sugar, cholesterol

- oregano: antioxidant, anti-inflammatory, antibacterial

- cumin: detoxification

- garlic: antibiotic, anticancer, lowering cholesterol and blood pressure

- ginger: anti-nausea, anti-oxidant, anti-inflammatory

- thyme: anticancer properties

- turmeric: anti-inflammatory, anticancer (Pratt and Kolberg 2009)

While the list of important spices is much longer, the point is to think of your spice cabinet as a natural-food medicine cabinet. Seasoning to taste is generally adequate, though some of these spices—for example, garlic, ginger, and turmeric—are available in supplement form from your health-food store.

THE SUPERFOODS Rx SUPERHEALTH FOOD PYRAMID

In case you didn't find a pyramid you really liked during the pyramid exercise in chapter 2, take a look at the SuperFoodsRx SuperHealth Food Pyramid (figure 2). This pyramid stands the usual pyramid on its end, making it easier to read from top to bottom.

SuperHealth Food Pyramid from Pratt and Kolberg (2009)

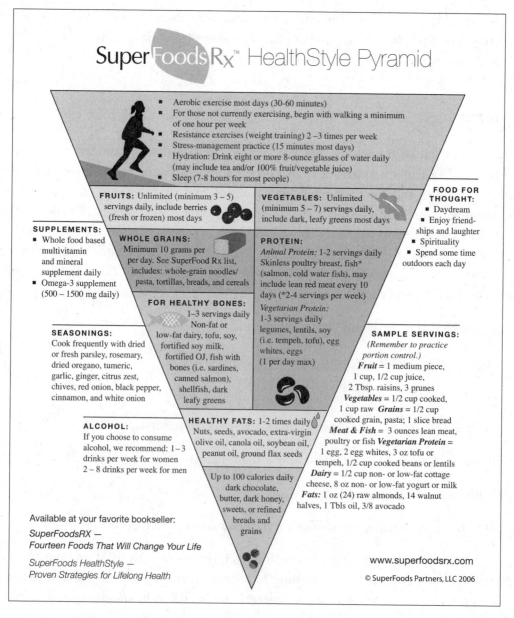

SuperFoodsRx™ HealthStyle Pyramid

- Aerobic exercise most days (30-60 minutes)
- For those not currently exercising, begin with walking a minimum of one hour per week
- Resistance exercises (weight training) 2–3 times per week
- Stress-management practice (15 minutes most days)
- Hydration: Drink eight or more 8-ounce glasses of water daily (may include tea and/or 100% fruit/vegetable juice)
- Sleep (7-8 hours for most people)

FRUITS: Unlimited (minimum 3 – 5) servings daily, include berries (fresh or frozen) most days

VEGETABLES: Unlimited (minimum 5 – 7) servings daily, include dark, leafy greens most days

FOOD FOR THOUGHT:
- Daydream
- Enjoy friend-ships and laughter
- Spirituality
- Spend some time outdoors each day

SUPPLEMENTS:
- Whole food based multivitamin and mineral supplement daily
- Omega-3 supplement (500 – 1500 mg daily)

WHOLE GRAINS: Minimum 10 grams per per day. See SuperFood Rx list, includes: whole-grain noodles/ pasta, tortillas, breads, and cereals

PROTEIN:
Animal Protein: 1-2 servings daily Skinless poultry breast, fish* (salmon, cold water fish), may include lean red meat every 10 days (*2-4 servings per week)
Vegetarian Protein: 1-3 servings daily legumes, lentils, soy (i.e. tempeh, tofu), egg whites, eggs (1 per day max)

FOR HEALTHY BONES: 1–3 servings daily Non-fat or low-fat dairy, tofu, soy, fortified soy milk, fortified OJ, fish with bones (i.e. sardines, canned salmon), shellfish, dark leafy greens

SEASONINGS: Cook frequently with dried or fresh parsley, rosemary, dried oregano, tumeric, garlic, ginger, citrus zest, chives, red onion, black pepper, cinnamon, and white onion

SAMPLE SERVINGS:
(Remember to practice portion control.)
Fruit = 1 medium piece, 1 cup, 1/2 cup juice, 2 Tbsp. raisins, 3 prunes
Vegetables = 1/2 cup cooked, 1 cup raw *Grains* = 1/2 cup cooked grain, pasta; 1 slice bread
Meat & Fish = 3 ounces lean meat, poultry or fish *Vegetarian Protein* = 1 egg, 2 egg whites, 3 oz tofu or tempeh, 1/2 cup cooked beans or lentils
Dairy = 1/2 cup non- or low-fat cottage cheese, 8 oz non- or low-fat yogurt or milk
Fats: 1 oz (24) raw almonds, 14 walnut halves, 1 Tbls oil, 3/8 avocado

ALCOHOL: If you choose to consume alcohol, we recommend: 1–3 drinks per week for women 2 – 8 drinks per week for men

HEALTHY FATS: 1-2 times daily Nuts, seeds, avocado, extra-virgin olive oil, canola oil, soybean oil, peanut oil, ground flax seeds

Up to 100 calories daily dark chocolate, butter, dark honey, sweets, or refined breads and grains

Available at your favorite bookseller:
SuperFoodsRX — Fourteen Foods That Will Change Your Life
SuperFoods HealthStyle — Proven Strategies for Lifelong Health

www.superfoodsrx.com

© SuperFoods Partners, LLC 2006

FIGURE 2: SuperFoodsrx SuperHealth Food Pyramid

The next exercise will help you identify the degree to which SuperFoods are already a part of your diet and discover how you might expand their presence.

EXERCISE: EATING MORE SUPERFOODS

Use the following worksheet to figure out how many SuperFoods you typically eat. The fourteen SuperFoods appear in a column on the left. In the boxes to the right, record how many servings of these SuperFoods and their sidekicks you have eaten over each of the past three days. Enter your three-day total for each SuperFood in the column on the right. For example, if you have had whole-grain cereal three times in the past three days, plus whole-grain bread for lunch sandwiches twice, and whole-grain brown rice for dinner twice, that's seven servings of "oats." Add the numbers in the column on the right to discover your grand total of SuperFood servings.

You wouldn't want to stack all your SuperFoods into one group, but over three days, you can sample some from most or even all the groups. If you are on the low side, start by changing how you shop.

EXERCISE: KEEP A SUPERFOODS SHOPPING LIST

Include on your shopping list at least one selection from each of the fourteen SuperFoods or sidekicks. Healthier eating usually requires you to add foods that may not be part of your customary diet. Look particularly at foods that you tend not to eat as much of, such as soy, skinless turkey breast, or pumpkin, and try adding one or two items you normally wouldn't buy or cook. Expand your list once a month. At the end of the year, your cart will be a rainbow of color, and your diet will have shifted to SuperFoods.

Don't worry if some of these foods are new to your diet. Try them out and you will find them delicious, nutritious, and easy to add to your lifestyle. Balance high-calorie items like salmon or nuts with fruits, veggies, and low-glycemic grains and beans. Portion control is essential. Note that a healthy portion of dense items like nuts would be a handful, whereas a healthy portion of veggies and fruits would be the size of a tennis ball. The standard dish portion for protein is about the size of a deck of cards, around four ounces of turkey, salmon, tuna, chicken, beans, and so on. If you like to eat out, remember that restaurant meals often contain several times these portions, so get used to taking home food. Split meals with family members to reduce the calories and to control portions.

SUPERFOOD THREE-DAY LOG

SuperFood	Day 1	Day 2	Day 3	Total Servings
Beans				
Blueberries				
Broccoli				
Oats				
Oranges				
Pumpkin				
Wild salmon				
Soy				
Spinach				
Tea				
Tomatoes				
Turkey breast				
Walnuts				
Yogurt				

Grand total SuperFood servings: _____

Scoring:

27 or higher = excellent (you ate three or more SuperFoods per meal)

9 to 18 = needs improvement (definitely on the low side: only one to two SuperFoods per meal)

less than 9 = time to revise your diet (you are likely eating a lot of unhealthy foods instead of SuperFoods)

OBESITY RISK REDUCTION

Obesity is now epidemic in the United States, so I remind you of the risks to your overall health of having all that pro-inflammatory fat around your waist. While people are always looking at quick fixes to reduce weight and improve their health, the following SuperFoods you are adding to your diet can help reduce obesity risk:

- The vitamin C in oranges and other citrus improves the efficiency of burning fat cells (Johnston 2005).

- Omega-3 fatty acids in fish reduce inflammation, which affects fat distribution as well as production of leptin, a fat-producing hormone (Hill et al. 2007).

- The calcium in yogurt and kefir promotes weight loss (Zemel 2005).

- The fiber in beans, broccoli, whole grains, and pumpkin increases satiety, slows sugar absorption, decreases food cravings, and improves gut *motility* (activity) and absorption.

- Turkey, soy, and salmon are quite low in saturated fats.

- Nuts, though high in calories, suppress appetite, reduce fat absorption, improve insulin control, and decrease inflammation, all of which helps with weight control (Rajaram and Sabaté 2006).

- Snacks or meal portions of spinach, broccoli, avocado, berries, tomatoes, and apples are good for you and much lower in calories than a soda or candy bar, reducing calorie intake substantially between meals.

- Green or black tea is *thermogenic*, meaning it helps your body burn calories (Shixian et al. 2007).

See the resources at the back of the book for some excellent recipes for improving your digestive and overall wellness.

SUPERSIZE?

While almost nobody actually eats fast food every day for a month, drive-thru meals are a major part of the American culture. Eating out can be a risk to your waistline and health because of large portion sizes and, depending on your choices, the excess salt, saturated fats, and high-calorie, low-nutrient value foods.

EXERCISE: FAST-FOOD SURVEY

Answer the following questions to do a quick review of your fast-food intake.

1. How many times have you or your family picked up food through a window in the past two weeks?

2. How many times did you eat at a restaurant?

3. How often did you prepare, cook, and eat a meal in your home?

Look at your answers. There is nothing inherently wrong with eating out, but it has some risks. While fast-food restaurants are now offering more healthful choices, such as grilled chicken, salads, and fruits, you still need to be cautious about calorie counts and amounts of fat when you eat out.

The ease, convenience, sociability, and other aspects of eating are often factors in choosing outside dining. Nonetheless, you can rediscover the joys of cooking and eating at home as you add more SuperFoods to your diet. It's a fun, healthy, and thrifty choice.

CONCLUSION

Dr. Pratt's work has been a wonderful example of simplifying applied nutrition for digestive health and reduction of risk from many common diseases. This chapter is largely based on his books *SuperFoods Rx: Fourteen Foods That Will Change Your Life* (with Kathy Matthews; Harper, 2006); *SuperFoods Healthstyle: Simple Changes to Get the Most Out of Life for the Rest of Your Life* (with Kathy Matthews; Harper, 2006); *Superhealth: Six Simple Steps, Six Easy Weeks, One Longer, Healthier Life* (with Sharyn Kolberg; Signet, 2010); *The SuperFoods Rx Diet: Lose Weight with the Power of SuperNutrients* (with Wendy Bazilian and Kathy Matthews; Rodale, 2008). I highly recommend all four of them.

The SuperFoods plan is healthful, sustainable, and easily adaptable to your lifestyle. Your new awareness of just what is a good mix of healthy foods will bring dividends for your health and that of your family for years to come.

CHAPTER 5

IMMUNITY AND THE GUT

HOW YOU CAN KEEP YOUR GUT IN GOOD HEALTH

When most people think of the immune system, they think of lymph glands in the neck and under the arms, the tonsils and adenoids, white blood cells, and perhaps the liver and spleen. However, the body's biggest collection of immune cells is in the gut (Takahashi and Kiyono 1999). This chapter will show you how to keep your whole body healthy by keeping your gut healthy.

HOW YOUR GUT PROTECTS YOU

Lymph tissue in the gut is composed of specialized clusters of cells, or Peyer's patches, as well as individual cells within the gut tissue and appendix. These cells secrete antibodies, such as immunoglobulin A (IgA), which is our first line of immune defense in the gut as well as in the mouth, nose, and throat.

What is it, exactly, that this mass of cells is protecting you against? The gut is heavily populated with bacteria and not all of them friendly. The gut antibodies, along with friendly bacteria, such as the probiotics, keep these unfriendly bacteria from overpopulating and invading your bloodstream. To get a sense of the size of this task, realize that one teaspoon of fluid in the small intestine can easily contain millions of bacteria, and the same amount of fluid in the colon holds a trillion or more.

Additionally, each of us sends down the food tube an estimated 25 to 30 tons of food plus liquids over the course of a lifetime, all of which has to be monitored for bacteria, viruses, and other types of antigens, toxins, and food allergens (see chapter 6). A breakdown in this process can result in immune weakness. It can also cause hyperimmune responses resulting in food allergy, inflammation, or autoimmune disease, in which the immune system attacks the body. Contributing to any of these is a condition called *leaky gut syndrome*, which is the focus of this chapter.

LEAKY GUT

Imagine stretching out a thirty-foot garden hose in your backyard. That's approximately the length of your small and large intestine combined. When you turn the hose on, the water comes right out the other end. Now, imagine running over the hose repeatedly with a lawnmower or some other power tool, leaving numerous holes, gashes, and slices. What happens now when you turn on the water? It would be leaking, spraying, and dribbling all along the hose, although some water would still be coming out the other end.

That simple backyard analogy gives you a sense of how a leak or multiple leaks in a long tube like your gut can have a major effect on its form and function. In the case of the body, many things can affect the gut, causing it to leak and damaging its important function as an absorptive, semipermeable barrier and a part of our immune surveillance.

The following conditions, diseases, and related treatments may cause damage to gut integrity (Jones and Quinn 2005):

- alcoholism

- asthma

- cancer and cancer treatments such as chemo and radiation

- celiac disease, or gluten intolerance

- cirrhosis

- drugs, nonsteroidal anti-inflammatories (ibuprofen), antibiotics, steroids

- dysbiosis (an imbalance in types of gut bacteria)

- excessive intake of simple sugars

- eczema

- exposure to whole foods before age four months

- food allergies

- infections (bacterial, viral, parasites, HIV)

- inflammatory bowel disease (Crohn's disease, ulcerative colitis)

- inflammatory joint disease

- lactose intolerance

- malnutrition

- pancreatic insufficiency

- premature birth

- psoriasis

- stress

- trauma

Essentially, these conditions and a number of others can open up the lining of the gut and cause it to be *hyperpermeable* to larger food particles, intact proteins, and toxins that should not be entering the bloodstream directly. This triggers an immune or inflammatory process that can contribute to, cause, or worsen the development of a long list of problems: ADHD, chronic fatigue, various types of arthritis, inflammatory and irritable bowel disease, multiple chemical sensitivities, skin problems, food allergies, liver problems, and more (Hijazi et al. 2004; Wilson et al. 2003).

DIAGNOSING LEAKY GUT

If you suffer from some of these symptoms, you may be experiencing the clinical effects of leaky gut. The following quiz can help you determine if you have leaky gut.

DO YOU HAVE LEAKY GUT?

Place a check mark next to any of the following conditions that reflect your experience, and then add up the number that you checked to determine your total score:

_____ You are prone to colds and other types of infections.

_____ When you get an infection, it takes longer than average to heal.

_____ If you get a wound or other skin injury, it takes a long time to heal.

_____ You have to take antibiotics several times a year.

_____ You take or have taken steroids or nonsteroidal anti-inflammatory drugs in the past year.

_____ You have had radiation or chemotherapy.

_____ You drink alcohol heavily (more than three drinks a day for women, four for men).

_____ You have chronic fatigue.

_____ You have frequent low-grade fevers.

_____ You have multiple joint aches.

_____ You have frequent diarrhea.

_____ You have frequent gastrointestinal infections.

_____ You are under chronic stress.

_____ You eat a lot of simple sugars or drink sugary sodas regularly.

_____ You have food allergies.

_____ You are malnourished due to caloric deprivation, an eating disorder, or poor choice of foods.

Your total score: _____

Scoring:

1 to 5 = some immune impairment and possible leaky gut

5 to 10 = moderate immune impairment and significant risk of leaky gut

Greater than 10 = high level of immune impairment and likely leaky gut

Quiz adapted from the Institute for Functional Medicine

HOW TO TREAT LEAKY GUT

If you suspect that you do have leaky gut, what do you do about it? You can't simply throw out your gut and replace it with a new one, as if it were a leaky garden hose. So how do you minimize the impact on your health or prevent leaky gut from happening in the first place? It's best to approach this problem using the four Rs of functional medicine: remove, replace, reinoculate, and repair (Jones and Quinn 2005). These are explained below.

Remove

To *remove* means to eliminate the cause of the problem. As you review what may be damaging your gut integrity, some obvious items to remove might be certain foods to which you are allergic or hypersensitive, alcohol, toxins in the water or food you consume, and infections in the stomach or gut. Some examples of infections would be an infection with the bacteria *Helicobacter pylori*, which is associated with ulcers and gastritis, or a lower GI infection with a parasite like *Giardia* or *E. coli*, both of which are causes of waterborne and so-called traveler's diarrhea. You will need medical attention and often medication to resolve either acute or chronic infections, which can cause burning, bloating, cramps, diarrhea, and gas. You will also want to remove, to the degree possible, certain drugs that irritate the gut, overly suppress acid, and otherwise damage the mucosal surfaces (see chapter 10). Dealing with stress more effectively can be a big help. For this, I highly recommend *The Relaxation and Stress Reduction Workbook* (see Resources) and chapter 8.

Replace

To *replace* what's missing, you can help the digestive system have what it needs to get well again. This might take the form of supplementing certain digestive enzymes that may be missing or inadequate, such as pancreatic enzymes or other enzymes that break down starch, carbohydrates, milk sugars, proteins, or fats. Low stomach acid can deliver incompletely digested foods that challenge the downstream immune system, so replacing with hydrochloric acid tablets can help with food allergies and more. See chapter 9 for guidance here.

Reinoculate

You can *reinoculate* your gut by introducing healthful bacteria, prebiotics, probiotics, and synbiotics, a mixture of prebiotics and probiotics (see chapter 3), particularly after a treatment with powerful drugs like chemotherapy, steroids, or antibiotics. These drugs can leave the immune system vulnerable, as the resulting dysbiosis affects the biofilms and the protective effects of healthy bacteria that interact with the cells lining the gut. If you have been on a course of anti-biotics, you may want to try a mixture of probiotics at sufficient doses of 10 to 30 billion units a day. Exactly what mix of bacteria and length of treatment is inconclusive from research studies, but I usually recommend these healthy bacteria for two to four weeks at a minimum in preventing or treating suspected dysbiosis.

Repair

Repair is the fourth step in the four Rs program, and you can accomplish it through a variety of methods, depending on the initial problem. Certain supplements can help support the intestinal cells and help them recover from damage. Among these are fish oil, pantothenic acid, zinc, and glutamine. Fish oil is one form of essential fatty acid useful for reducing gut inflammation; pantothenic acid is a B-type vitamin that concentrates in the gut and supports normal mucosal function and healing in colitis. Certain conditions like inflammatory bowel disease deplete zinc, which further diminishes immunity and wound healing, unless provided for in the repair process. Keep in mind that many essential nutrients can be obtained in food sources, particularly SuperFoods, and do not necessarily require a supplement or a pill. See chapter 9 for details on how to do this, or consult with an integrative health practitioner.

CONCLUSION

Certain medical conditions can damage your immune system through their activity in the gut and their impact on its permeability. In other cases, the leaky gut is an upstream cause of these conditions. As a result, it is sometimes difficult to determine the cause of leaky gut: was it the anti-inflammatory or steroid drug used to treat a joint problem, or did the problem start before that? It is important to think of this as a reciprocal process in which cause and effect may blur. Ultimately, treating the root cause in the gut can help the systemic disease as much or more than the treatment of its symptoms. The next two chapters cover the issues of food sensitivities and gut inflammation, which are related to this complex chain of events.

CHAPTER 6

WHAT YOU ARE EATING
MAY BE EATING YOU

FOOD ALLERGIES
AND SENSITIVITIES

Do you have food allergies? How would you know? Many subtle symptoms may be due to reactions to foods, either frank allergic reactions or hypersensitivity to a food. The most common foods responsible for a true food allergy related to reactions in the immune system are wheat, dairy, eggs, peanuts, soy, shellfish, fish, and tree nuts. You may want to consider food allergy as a cause for any unexplained medical symptoms. You are more likely at risk if you have other allergies like asthma, hay fever, eczema, or drug allergies, or if you have a family history of allergies. Symptoms can be extremely wide ranging, and though food allergy starts in the gut, it can and does affect nearly every body system.

TYPES OF FOOD ALLERGY

There are two basic types of food allergy. They each create the potential for certain reactions. Some reactions are rapid and serious and, in rare cases, even fatal. Other reactions are more subtle and slower to present, though they can also be quite troublesome.

Rapid Onset

If you eat a certain food, say shrimp or peanuts, and you have an immediate reaction of shortness of breath, hives, and/or swelling of the throat, you are experiencing a rapid *IgE-mediated* (a kind of immune molecule) immediate hypersensitivity reaction. You can remember IgE as in E for *emergency*. This allergic reaction typically occurs within twenty minutes of exposure to a food, though it may take up to two hours, and resolves within four to twelve hours. This reaction is *repetitive* in that it occurs whenever you eat the suspect food. If you have an IgE-mediated food allergy, you probably have an aversion to the food that triggers your reaction.

IgE-mediated food allergies may be accompanied by the following symptoms:

- rapid onset of symptoms, with brief duration

- anaphylaxis (shock resulting from intake of a food or drug)

- itchy rash or flushing

- angioedema (diffuse swelling of lips, tongue, face, and/or body)

- asthma or wheezing

- nausea

- abdominal cramps

- diarrhea

- light-headedness or fainting

- chronic sinusitis

- unexplained hives, rash, or other dermatological symptoms

Any of the above symptoms may be associated with a serious food allergy, but if you have experienced a rapid onset of symptoms, anaphylaxis, itchy rash or flushing, and angioedema after ingesting a particular food, it is highly likely that you have this kind of IgE-mediated allergy. To be safe, check with an allergist. Blood and skin tests can help your physician and you determine for sure if certain foods are causing serious reactions. Until then, you ought to stay away from any food that you suspect is a problem.

With this kind of food allergy, you may need to carry an epinephrine injection pen (Epi-Pen) with you to manage emergency reactions. Having this medication on you can be the difference between life and death. A colleague who was violently allergic to mushrooms was once accidentally served some in her restaurant meal and had an immediate reaction of throat swelling and difficulty breathing. She was lucky to be carrying an Epi-Pen and antihistamines for just such an event.

It is estimated that this kind of food allergy afflicts 4 percent of the U.S. population, or 12 million people, and it is increasingly prevalent among children. In fact, food allergies in general in children have risen 18 percent in the past decade (Lack 2008). Peanut allergy, which doubled during the five-year period ending in 2002, can be a serious problem indeed, where even inhaling peanut aroma can trigger a severe attack. When in doubt, get a medical consultation regarding this kind of severe food allergy.

Slow Onset

Other symptoms may be the result of *IgG-mediated* (another immune molecule) reactions and are subtler and longer term in nature. These allergic reactions are typically harder to diagnose and treat since your reaction to a particular food can be delayed twelve to twenty-four hours or even longer. You can remember IgG as in G for *gradual*. Both GI and non-GI-related conditions may be related to a food allergy/sensitivity. Some foods cause reactions when eaten with other foods, such as fish and dairy, the so-called coallergy reaction.

What causes you to develop this kind of allergy may be hard to pinpoint, but the following conditions are considered culprits: formula instead of breast feeding as an infant; a diet heavy in high-glycemic foods; increased gut permeability (leaky gut); gut dysbiosis; and even lack of exposure to dirt and germs early in life. Apparently, it is good for kids to consume a certain amount of dirt, germs, and other things we think of as less than clean, for this exposure helps their immune systems develop adequately. A limited exposure of the immune system to foreign substances seems to cause the body to fail to recognize them later in life, which promotes an allergic reaction (Matsui et al. 2004).

The following symptoms may be related to chronic IgG-mediated food allergies:

General: fatigue and general malaise; sleep disturbances

Mental/neurological: cognition changes (brain fog); anxiety; depression; attention deficit disorder; migraine headache

Infectious/allergic: nasal congestion/chronic sinusitis; recurrent ear infections; vertigo or dizziness; sore throat; allergic nose rub; dark circles under the eyes (allergic shiners); asthma

Gastrointestinal: esophageal discomfort (heartburn, spasms); abdominal pain; diarrhea or constipation

Dermatological: chronic hives; eczema

Genitourinary: urinary symptoms (infection, burning); recurrent vaginitis

Musculoskeletal/extremities: arthritis; muscle soreness; mild edema (evidenced by sock marks, underwear marks)

Hematological/lymphatic: enlarged lymph nodes; easy bruising

Obviously, such a long list of symptoms can make it hard to determine if a particular food, food group, or combination of foods is triggering an IgG immune-related food allergy. Food allergy like this is not just a discrete pathological process like, say, strep throat or pneumonia, but results in a broad immune-mediated inflammatory response in the gut. A leaky, inflamed, allergic gut activates immune complexes that circulate in the blood throughout the rest of the body and wreak damage far from the original site of the allergic reaction. To help you understand how this kind of reaction can occur, here is a closer look at a specific kind of food sensitivity, the reaction to gluten.

GLUTEN INTOLERANCE: A COMMON BUT UNDERDIAGNOSED PROBLEM

A common and potentially serious food allergy problem is *gluten intolerance*. Gluten is a form of protein found in wheat and other grains. This condition is both an IgG-mediated allergy and also an *IgA-mediated* allergy (IgA is an immunoglobulin that is secreted on the surface of mucosal tissues). Gluten intolerance and its most severe form, celiac disease, can present with many subtle signs and symptoms, which can delay diagnosis for up to a decade or more. By this time, people have suffered from a variety of symptoms—diarrhea, malabsorption, osteoporosis, arthritis, fatigue, systemic inflammation, anemia, diabetes, depression, poor pregnancy outcomes, and immune problems—triggered by eating food that contains gluten. The only really effective treatment for this condition is a lifelong dietary abstinence from all foods containing gluten. Specialized testing including blood work and gut tissue biopsy are necessary for a complete workup (Fasano 2009).

In fact, probiotics, the health-promoting bacteria discussed in chapter 3, may be highly influential in whether you are able to tolerate gluten or other foods. This is because probiotics help in processes of absorption, immune regulation, and recognition of foreign substances and can actually reduce your risk of reacting to gluten. The mix of foods you take in can also affect this process, so eating foods high in sugars and fats can alter your gut bacteria and increase a tendency to food allergy and its GI and systemic symptoms (Preidis and Versalovic 2009; De Palma et al. 2009). Some people have milder forms of gluten and other food sensitivities, leading to such vague symptoms as fatigue, aching of the joints and muscles, brain fog (a state of impaired concentration, memory, and general awareness), gastrointestinal distress, skin rash, and asthma. If you have such symptoms, at least consider gluten to be a possible factor. For more information, check out the user-friendly website of the nonprofit National Foundation for Celiac Awareness (see resources).

The functional-medicine approach is to investigate the full spectrum of the digestive process to assess if there is any problem in digestion, absorption, elimination, and microbiota balance and to consider allergic reaction, hypersensitivity, or any other factors that could be contributing to health problems.

HYPERSENSITIVITY AND OTHER DIGESTIVE PROBLEMS

Perhaps you are not frankly allergic to foods or food groups but can't digest them well, or they lead to other symptoms in your body. These symptoms can be in the gut, such as gas, cramping, indigestion, irritable bowel, nausea, recurrent canker sores, ulcers, inflammatory bowel disease, celiac disease, or chronic diarrhea. As in immune-related food allergy, reactions outside the gut can also occur in either contributing to or worsening of autoimmune diseases like lupus and rheumatoid arthritis; neurological symptoms including depression, cognitive/thinking dysfunction, brain fog, hyperactivity, or headaches; unexplained hives or rashes; unexplained fatigue, joint pain, or muscle pain; and irritable bladder.

You may also react to other foods that you aren't really allergic to but that you lack the *enzyme* (a chemical to stimulate the digestive process) to digest. A common example of this is *lactose intolerance,* in which the enzyme lactase is missing so that you cannot tolerate dairy products, except perhaps for yogurt, in which bacteria start the process of digestion of *lactose* (milk sugar) during the preparation process. If you suspect that you have a dairy allergy because of symptoms after consuming milk products, you may in fact be experiencing not an allergy but lactase deficiency. Adding lactase from such products as Lactaid or lactase capsules will help solve this food intolerance problem. You can also choose lactose-free foods like soymilk or soy yogurt.

In addition, people deficient in certain digestive enzymes or chemicals like hydrochloric acid in the stomach or pancreatic enzymes such as *protease* (which breaks down protein), *lipase* (which breaks down fat), and *amylase* (which breaks down carbohydrates) may be more prone to food allergy, as foods are not broken down to their elemental components before being presented to the downstream gut. For further discussion of what you can do to compensate for these deficiencies, see chapter 9.

SELF-DIAGNOSIS BY RECORDING AND MANIPULATING YOUR DIET

There are two basic methods you can use to figure out for yourself if what you're eating is part of your health problems. Using a food elimination diet and reintroduction process is one method (see chapter 11). Keeping a food diary and symptom log is another.

THREE-DAY DIET DIARY AND SYMPTOM LOG

Complete this diary and symptom log for three consecutive days (one day should be a weekend day). It is important to keep an accurate record of your usual food and beverage intake, along with any associated symptoms, using the following instructions:

1. Record information as soon as possible after eating.

2. Maintain your usual eating behavior at this time unless your doctor advises you to change it. The purpose of this food record is to analyze your present eating habits.

3. Describe the food or beverage consumed, and be specific: for example, milk (whole, 2 percent, or nonfat); toast (whole wheat, white, buttered); chicken (fried, baked, breaded).

4. Record the amount of each food consumed using standard measurements as much as possible, such as eight ounces, half a cup, one teaspoon.

5. Include any added items: for example, tea with one teaspoon sugar, potato with two teaspoons butter.

6. Record all beverages, including water, in the Beverage column.

7. Record all bowel movements and their consistency (regular, loose, firm).

8. Record any physical symptoms you may experience during the three days and compare them to the food allergy/sensitivity symptoms listed earlier in the chapter.

9. Record any suspected food association.

THREE-DAY DIET DIARY

Date:

Time	Food	Amount	Time	Beverage	Amount
_____	_____	_____	_____	_____	_____
_____	_____	_____	_____	_____	_____
_____	_____	_____	_____	_____	_____
_____	_____	_____	_____	_____	_____
_____	_____	_____	_____	_____	_____
_____	_____	_____	_____	_____	_____
_____	_____	_____	_____	_____	_____
_____	_____	_____	_____	_____	_____
_____	_____	_____	_____	_____	_____
_____	_____	_____	_____	_____	_____
_____	_____	_____	_____	_____	_____

Bowel Movements

Time	Consistency
_____	_____
_____	_____
_____	_____
_____	_____
_____	_____

SYMPTOM LOG

Time/Date	Symptoms (New reaction or worsening of existing condition)	Suspected Food Association

Three-day diet diary and symptom log adapted from the Institute for Functional Medicine

If you have noted one or more symptoms occurring or worsening during the three days that you are doing this exercise, you ought to at least consider potential food-related problems. Even if there is another well-diagnosed reason for the symptom or it is chronic, such detective work can help you determine if a certain food type is making your symptoms worse. For example, some kinds of arthritis may become worse when you eat certain types of foods, such as those containing gluten, or nightshade family plants like tomatoes, eggplant, and white potatoes.

If you feel as a result of the information presented in this chapter or as a result of your completing this food diary and symptom log that you are possibly suffering from food-related problems, the next step is a more precise diagnosis.

Your physician can help diagnose food allergies through blood and skin testing; such tests provide information that is highly sensitive in detecting certain food allergies and can be helpful particularly for the dangerous IgE-mediated conditions. However, these tests are not as useful or sensitive for IgG-mediated or food-sensitivity conditions. In fact, positive results from these tests may not be clinically important. More important is determining exactly how your body reacts to a given food.

One of the very best methods is the highly useful therapeutic and diagnostic tool known as the elimination diet. If you have food allergies or sensitivities, this diet will make you feel better as you remove foods that are causing trouble. You follow the elimination diet for three weeks and then gradually reintroduce the foods you have eliminated. As you reintroduce these foods, one at a time, and experience familiar symptoms, you can diagnose the culprit food. If you think that you could benefit from this process, see chapter 11 for more details.

CONCLUSION

A holistic approach to your overall gut health, as well as the rest of your body, ought to start with a review of your diet. If you have a strong family or personal history of allergies to drugs or other substances, hay fever, asthma, or atopic eczema, you are likely at higher risk for food-related allergy. Children who were bottle-fed rather than breast-fed are also at higher risk.

Because conventional allergy testing for food is often inconclusive or nonspecific, other more functional approaches can be helpful to your gut's health and healing.

Chapter 7

The Anti-Inflammatory Diet

Healing Your Gut, Joints, Blood Vessels, Brain, Heart, and More

Inflammation is not always a bad thing. *Acute inflammation* is a normal bodily and gut process, helping to heal infections, injuries, and other insults to the system. Picture yourself getting a splinter in your finger and leaving it there for a while. You will observe the cardinal manifestations of inflammation: redness (*rubor*), heat (*calor*), swelling (*tumor*), and pain (*dolor*), as described in both English and Latin for every medical student. This is the typical acute inflammatory process. Note that after the splinter is removed, the inflammation dies down, and your finger feels better as the wound generally heals without any difficulty. After the initiating event, the body's proinflammatory system activates cellular destruction. This then is countered by an anti-inflammatory healing response leading to cellular repair and regeneration.

So far, so good. This is the normal chain of events as your body heals the usual cuts, bruises, and infections of daily life. The persistence of inflammation, however, is a major health risk for many conditions.

This chapter deals with *silent inflammation*, which, unlike acute inflammation, you don't usually even notice. It is a chronic process that goes on for years, even decades, generally without our awareness of it. It is recognized as a common pathway to many chronic afflictions and diseases, including coronary artery disease, hypertension, and diabetes, and is now considered a likely contributing factor to neurodegenerative diseases, like Alzheimer's disease and Parkinsonism, and even obesity.

Silent inflammation may affect appearance, accelerating aging, wrinkling skin, and causing bone deterioration, hormonal changes, and more. These roles of inflammation have been recognized in cutting-edge clinical science in functional and integrative medicine for many years. They are now coming to be accepted by conventional physicians and researchers as well.

THE MOUTH: A SOURCE OF INFLAMMATION

The start of the gut is the mouth, so it may not be surprising to learn that the mouth is a source of inflammation. *Gingivitis*, or inflammation of the gums, may affect heart health (Hujoel et al. 2000), increase stroke risk (Scannapieco, Bush, and Paju 2003), and even be related to risks for diabetes (Taylor 2001) and obesity (Pischon et al. 2007). Insurance companies recognize that good oral hygiene is necessary to overall health when they pay for regular dental cleaning. Daily hygiene through regular brushing and flossing is essential to protect against cavities, loss of teeth from gum disease, and the systemic impacts of gum inflammation elsewhere. It helps in your social space, too, to have a nice smile and good breath.

THE PHYSIOLOGY OF INFLAMMATION

Inflammation is a complex orchestration of events in the body mediated by chemical substances that simultaneously stimulate the processes of injury and repair. Initiating events such as infections and injuries prompt acute inflammation and rubor, calor, tumor, and dolor. Such inflammation can easily become chronic and is initiated and then potentially sustained by a variety of factors, many of which are modifiable through lifestyle and dietary changes. This kind of inflammation can result in damage to a blood vessel wall, leading to rupture of an atherosclerotic plaque, a buildup in cholesterol in the blood vessel wall.

Going to Waist

A large waist circumference can lead to chronic inflammation and is a risk factor for disease. Increased circumference results from a buildup of fat in the abdominal cavity. This excess fat acts like a separate organ. It stores fat and toxins soluble in fat and is a major source of proinflammatory substances released into the body, including cytokines, eicosanoids, leukotrienes, and other chemicals that stimulate inflammation (Lemieux et al. 2001).

MEASURING YOUR WAIST

Measure your waist circumference:

1. Stand up straight and relax.

2. Pull down the top of your underwear to below waist level.

3. Locate your waist, at the top of the hipbone on the side and the crest of the iliac bone in the back. To find this bone, put your hands on your hips at the side of your body, extending the thumbs toward the center of your back.

4. Place measuring tape horizontally around your waist, snug but not pressing the skin.

5. Breathe in and out, measuring the waist at the end of expiration.

A waist circumference of over forty inches in men and over thirty-five inches in women is a marker of obesity and indicates an increased risk of metabolic syndrome (see next section). This risk gets higher the greater your body mass index (BMI).

CALCULATE YOUR BMI

Calculate your BMI using the following formula. Take your weight (in pounds) and multiply by 703; then divide that figure by your height (in inches) squared. Alternatively, it is much easier to use an online calculator or table to determine your BMI.

Use the following table to determine your weight classification:

Underweight: less than 18.5

Normal: 18.5 to 24.9

Overweight: 25.0 to 29.9

Obesity (class 1): 30.0 to 34.9

Obesity (class 2): 35.0 to 39.9

Extreme obesity: more than 40

BMI classifications from the National Heart, Lung, and Blood Institute *Obesity Education Initiative*, October 2000

When coupled with an above-normal BMI, a large waist circumference has been documented as a substantial risk for coronary artery disease, hypertension, diabetes, and other health problems. A large waistline is one of a group of risk factors for disease known as *metabolic syndrome.*

Metabolic Syndrome and Inflammation

Metabolic syndrome is characterized by an apple-shaped body typified by a larger amount of intra-abdominal fat. Criteria for the diagnosis include elevated blood pressure, abnormal fats (lipids like cholesterol and triglycerides), lower-than-normal HDL ("good") cholesterol level, and abnormally high blood sugar. Both insulin resistance and metabolic syndrome are associated with a diet high in refined carbohydrates and saturated fat, lack of exercise, obesity, and genetic factors. Excess insulin secretion is another initiating process for chronic inflammation.

WHAT YOU CAN DO TO REDUCE INFLAMMATION

The good news is that by making some dietary changes, you can significantly reduce or eliminate chronic inflammation and associated health risks. A quick food quiz can assess your diet from the perspective of being inflammatory or not.

HAVE YOU BEEN EATING INFLAMMATORY FOODS?

Take a snapshot of your last two days of meals to see whether the foods you've been eating are anti-inflammatory or proinflammatory. Check off the foods in the two columns that you have eaten in the past forty-eight hours.

Anti-Inflammatory Foods	Proinflammatory Foods
Fish, especially cold-water fish like salmon, sardines, tuna, mackerel, and herring, but also clams, oysters, tilapia, catfish, trout	White flours and grains with a high glycemic index, such as white bread, rice, crackers, baked goods, pasta
Free-range lean meats and wild game meats, such as turkey breast, skinless chicken, bison	Red meats with high saturated fat content
Flaxseed, other seeds and nuts	Dairy products and eggs (non–omega-3 enriched)
Green leafy vegetables, brightly colored vegetables (red, yellow, orange, purple)	High-fructose corn syrup contained in processed foods or beverages
Whole grains, high-fiber fruits, and vegetables	Foods containing trans-fatty acids
Tea, red wine	Partially hydrogenated oils such as corn, cottonseed, and sunflower oils
Olive oil	

The more items you checked off in the left column, the better. You'll notice that the anti-inflammatory diet looks a lot like the SuperFoods diet described in chapter 4.

Anti-Inflammatory Drugs, Anti-Inflammatory Foods, or Both?

Many contemporary drugs are designed to counter inflammation, including aspirin, nonsteroidal anti-inflammatory drugs (NSAIDs, like Motrin), prednisone and other steroids, colchicine for gout, COX-2 inhibitors (like Celebrex) for arthritis, sulfasalazine for inflammatory bowel disease, Singulair for asthma, and others.

These powerful drugs quiet inflammation by targeting inflammation that causes tissue destruction and illness. For example, the steroid drug prednisone may quiet inflammation but does not address the underlying cause. Such medications must be used with caution because they may have side effects, from weight gain and mood problems to blood clots, diarrhea, ulcers, high blood pressure, kidney and liver damage, and heart attack.

A number of foods and spices may have anti-inflammatory effects and influence the pathways with less toxicity than drugs. These include apples, onions, turmeric, soy, ginger, rosemary, red pepper, and anti-inflammatory medicinal herbs such as boswellia. Consuming these on a regular basis may reduce or eliminate the need for prescription drugs, saving money and avoiding the risks of medications. The amount will vary depending on your underlying conditions, but use the SuperFoods pyramid as a guide (see chapter 4). For herbs, use to taste when they have a culinary application or, if they are in capsule form, use guidelines included on the bottle. Usually a gram or two daily is an adequate anti-inflammatory dose of ginger, boswellia, and turmeric. Prescription drugs may be necessary and consultation with a physician required if dietary approaches are ineffective (Rakel and Rindfleisch 2005).

Fat Is Good! How Dietary Fats Can Affect Inflammation

Dietary fats contribute to the balance between the two bodily chemical processes of inflammation and anti-inflammation. Certain kinds of fat, like those from animal and dairy, contain the *omega-6 fatty acids*, which stimulate the inflammatory side of this cascade of events by producing a proinflammatory substance called *arachidonic acid*. This substance is changed into or stimulates other inflammatory chemicals. Such saturated fats turn on the inflammation cycle.

Other kinds of fats, derived from such foods as fish, green leafy vegetables, avocados, and nuts, competitively inhibit the enzyme that is involved in the inflammatory side of the cascade. This means that the metabolism pushes more of one kind of fat down the two pathways. If there are more of the healthier fats, they win out over the unhealthy ones. These healthier fats are called *omega-3 fatty acids*. Eating more foods containing such *essential fatty acids* (EFAs) reduces the production and release of arachidonic acid and other cytokine chemicals that lead to increased inflammation. Other healthy fats like olive and canola oil, *omega-9 fatty acids*, contribute to a better balance of anti-inflammatory fats to proinflammatory fats (Kris-Etherton et al. 2002).

Animal and dairy products may contain increased healthy fats when they are grass fed or free range or, as in the case of high omega-3 eggs, when feed is supplemented with fats such as flaxseed. Wild meats such as venison, buffalo, and elk are naturally grass fed, lower in saturated fats, and higher in healthy omega-3 fats than meats that are corn fattened in feedlots. Turkey breast and skinless chicken breast are other easily available sources of protein with less inflammatory mediators, especially when organic, hormone free, and/or free range.

GOOD FATS VS. BAD FATS

Researchers have calculated that the ideal ratio of inflammatory (or bad) fats to anti-inflammatory (good) fats in the diet is 4:1 or less. Unfortunately, the standard American diet contains a ratio of bad to good fats of 16:1 or even as high as 25:1 (Pischon et al. 2003). We have become a more obese society since the 1960s, when fat was considered to be an evil food. While there are many reasons for the obesity epidemic, including lack of exercise, types of food intake are as important as or even more important than calorie counts. Since those initial years when we became aware of the hazards of too much cholesterol, our society has increased its intake of carbohydrates (and calories), mostly high-glycemic carbohydrates, and other processed foods. This paranoia about fats has driven us to less healthy food choices.

True, cholesterol is a risk factor for heart disease, but as we discovered this, we neglected to note that healthy olive and fish oils in the typical Mediterranean diet actually reduce cardiac risk (de Lorgeril 1994). The Mediterranean diet pyramid (see Resources) significantly reduces the silent inflammation from our usual diet. It also helps reduce the risk of heart disease and other inflammation-related problems.

The following list of fats summarizes how different fats contained in food can have pro- or anti-inflammatory effects:

Saturated fats: Animal-based omega-6 producing proinflammatory arachidonic acid: beef and other animal fats; dairy products.

Polyunsaturated fats: Omega-3 and plant-based omega-6 producing anti-inflammatory mediators. Omega-3: alpha-linolenic acid (ALA) in legumes, leafy vegetables, flax, flaxseed, and canola oils; eicosopentanoic acid (EPA) in fish oil; docosahexanoic acid (DHA) in fish oil, breast milk. Omega-6: linoleic acid (LA) in vegetable oils, seeds, nuts; gamma-linolenic acid (GLA) in borage and primrose oil.

Monounsaturated fats: Anti-inflammatory omega-9 found in olive and canola oils.

Attaining a 4:1 ratio of bad to good fats generally requires at least 2.5 grams a day of omega-3 type fatty acids. Improving heart function, reducing pain, and addressing neurological or psychiatric disease requires even more omega-3s, up to 10 grams a day. These higher levels will require supplementation. For inflammatory conditions of the gut, use at least 2 grams of EFAs and double or triple that amount if there is no response.

Be sure to get good-quality fish oil if you are using supplements, so you eliminate or minimize the amount of mercury, dioxin, PCBs, and other contaminants that can be concentrated in fish. There are many high-quality products available, including Nordic Natural and Spectrum brands. Smaller fish, such as sardines and anchovies, which are lower down the food chain, and small tuna, like yellowfin or chunk light tuna, have lower levels of contaminants than larger fish. Avoid swordfish, tilefish, and bluefin or albacore tuna, or limit such intake to once a week or so.

FOOD AS INFORMATION

Food can be understood as calories made up of carbohydrates, protein, and fat, but food is also information. The food you put into your body can significantly alter the risks incurred for many diseases. This happens through signaling pathways within cells affected by the foods you eat. This concept has grown into the ever more sophisticated science of *nutrigenomics* (the science of how food modifies the activity of genes). Food choices give information to our metabolic system and modify chemical reactions like the inflammatory pathways already described. Further upstream in cellular biology, food can act by turning on or off certain genes responsible for essential processes: detoxification; *apoptosis*, or programmed cellular death, which prevents cancer from forming or spreading; and synthesis of essential proteins and immune elements. A recent report showed that a salad of raw vegetables and olive oil recommended in seventeenth-century Italy has been found to shut off *oncogenes*, or breast-cancer promoting genes (Colomer et al. 2008). Such factors help us understand the potential of food as a healing or disease-promoting choice in our lives. We have shown how food is anti-inflammatory and antioxidant. We now are beginning to recognize how food is also an *epi-genetic factor*, affecting the functions of our genes and creating conditions that reduce risks of cancer and other diseases.

Food Choices...What Should You Avoid?

Combining information gathered in recent clinical and nutritional studies, you can easily identify certain foods you ought to eat (see chapter 4) and those you need to avoid. You should try to avoid or reduce the following:

- trans-fatty acids (bad!)

- animal-based omega-6 fatty acids

- margarine

- corn oil, cottonseed oil, grapeseed oil, peanut oil, safflower oil, sesame oil, soybean oil, sunflower oil, partially hydrogenated oils

- crackers, pastries, chips, or any product with a long shelf life

Trans fats are particularly inflammatory, for we have no specific metabolic pathway to handle them. These fats are heated to a high temperature in the presence of a catalyst to twist certain chemical bonds, which renders them more stable on the shelf and less likely to become rancid. This may be good for food companies, but it's bad on our biology. As shown in figure 3, trans-fatty acids may compose as much as 2 to 3 percent of the American diet.

MAJOR FOOD SOURCES OF TRANS *FAT FOR AMERICAN ADULTS*
(AVERAGE DAILY TRANS FAT INTAKE IS 5.8 GRAMS OR 2-3 PERCENT OF CALORIES)

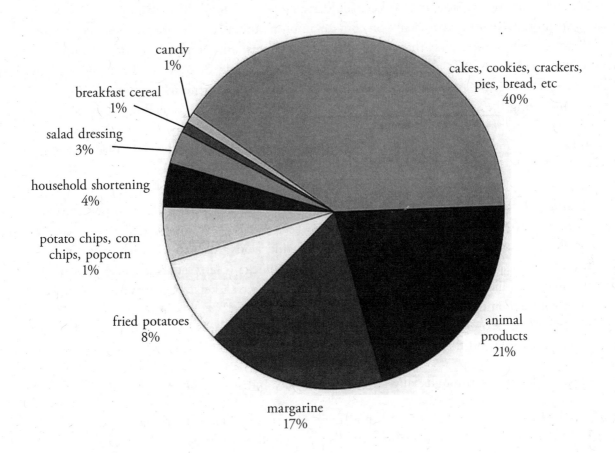

candy
1%

breakfast cereal
1%

salad dressing
3%

household shortening
4%

potato chips, corn
chips, popcorn
1%

fried potatoes
8%

cakes, cookies, crackers,
pies, bread, etc
40%

animal
products
21%

margarine
17%

Data from the U.S. Food and Drug Administration, July 2003

FIGURE 3: MAJOR FOOD SOURCES OF TRANS FAT FOR AMERICAN ADULTS

The percentage of trans fats in our diet is dropping as trans fats are increasingly regulated in restaurants and as food-labeling requirements have become stricter. Currently, any food with 0.5 percent or more trans fats must document this on the label. Note that if a label states "no trans fats," it may very well contain trans fats under the 0.5 percent limit, so be careful when you shop. If you want to reduce your intake of these unhealthy fats, look at figure 3 to see where you might cut down on trans-fatty foods in your diet.

So, What Should You Eat?

Perhaps the simplest advice is offered by Michael Pollan (2008). He recommends unprocessed, whole foods that your great-grandmother would recognize as a food. This means avoiding foods that have more than five ingredients or contain unpronounceable substances, foods containing high-fructose corn syrup, foods that make health-food claims, and processed food-like substances rather than real foods. We have no idea how the complex mix of food additives, with many new-to-nature molecules, affects our inflammatory pathways, our genomic expression, and their impact on setting the stage for disease. Pollan gives an example that is shocking. He describes a commercial white bread with over forty ingredients listed on the package. Grandma would have baked something made up of whole-grain flour, yeast, water, and a little salt, and called it "bread." I would call it healthy and delicious. This was a truly different bread from the one described previously!

Finding real food can be a challenge. Here are some strategies: grow your own food, eat wild game or fish, frequent local farmers' markets, and seek out organic foods. A diet of such real foods provides the fiber, phytonutrients, and low-glycemic foods that you need while helping you attain the proper anti-inflammatory mix of omega-3 to omega-6 fatty acids. Reduce your intake of processed food-like substances that weigh down the supermarket store shelves, your grocery cart, and your abdominal fat pad.

The following recommended lifestyle changes and strategies will help you reduce inflammation in your lifestyle and diet, moving in the right direction for your gut and overall health:

Lose fat. Burn calories through daily aerobic, resistance, and stretching exercise.

Eat small meals. Eat until you are full, not more. Use smaller plates. Have restaurant meals cut in half in the kitchen or at the table to take home. Avoid food after the dinner meal.

Have some protein at every meal. Reduce red meat and dairy. Avoid charred, overcooked foods. Vegetable protein such as soy and other beans is a good option.

Increase omega-3 fatty acids. Eat more cold-water fish, such as salmon, mackerel, sardines, herring, and tuna.

Cook with healthy fats. Emphasize omega-9 fatty acids like olive oil and canola oil for cooking, marinating, salad dressings, and dipping. Use hummus or olive-oil-based mayonnaise as a spread instead of butter.

Eat primarily fruits and vegetables. Increase the proportion of these important antioxidant, anti-inflammatory foods in your diet per meal and every day. Eat something green with every meal, maybe even at breakfast.

Exercise with a mixture of aerobic, resistance, flexibility, and balance activities. Set goals for thirty to sixty minutes daily using the FITT program: frequency (how often per week); intensity (low, moderate, heavy); type (aerobic, resistance, etc.); time (number of minutes/hours).

Quit smoking. Just do it! Use behavioral techniques (hypnosis), acupuncture, tobacco withdrawal patches, gum, smokeless cigarettes, or medication as needed.

Manage stress. Try relaxation exercises, such as meditation, biofeedback, deep breathing, imagery, autogenics, hypnosis, and mindfulness; use movement therapies, such as yoga or tai chi, or aerobics, like walking, swimming, or running; get social, relational, or community support; develop a spiritual practice; treat depression.

CONCLUSION

You can reduce your risk of many systemic conditions by using your gut as a source of healing. First recognize the difference between proinflammatory and anti-inflammatory foods and make well-considered choices to include less of one and more of the other as you shop, cook, or eat out. Eat well, enjoying the omnivorous life of healthy foods and healthy fats from both plant and animal sources, or, if you choose, go vegetarian. The key is to select the best food types and maintain the many aspects of a healthy lifestyle.

CHAPTER 8

GUT FEELINGS

HOW YOUR GUT AFFECTS AND IS AFFECTED BY YOUR EMOTIONS

This chapter explores how the gut affects and is affected by your emotional life. It includes a number of exercises to help you get in closer touch with your gut feelings and to cope with stress and distressing emotions.

You have no doubt heard such expressions as "I can't stomach him," "I've got a bad feeling in my gut about this," "She makes me want to puke," "My gut-level reaction to that is...," and so on. Where do these expressions come from?

Part of the answer may be that the GI tract is richly loaded with chemical receptors that affect not only digestion but also mood and feeling. It is densely populated with the kinds of cellular secretions (*serotonin*) present in the brain and central nervous system. Such serotonin-secreting nerve cells are the targets of antidepressant drugs known as selective serotonin reuptake inhibitors (SSRIs). Examples are drugs such as Prozac, Zoloft, Paxil, Celexa, and Effexor. Medical physiology research thus shows that some of the same mechanisms affecting the thoughts and emotions in the brain are involved in the gut, which is populated by similar cells secreting identical chemicals.

So the gut is a place where emotions, as well as food, are processed.

LINKING YOUR GUT TO YOUR EMOTIONS

In addition to the role of such neurochemicals, the gut is also under the strong influence of the vagus nerve, a major nerve that affects heart function as well. The vagus nerve is the "wandering" nerve (from the same Latin root from which we get words like "vagabond" and "vagrant"). It wanders through the head, neck, and chest and into the belly. The heart, as we well know, is also an organ of emotion and has been celebrated as such by poets, mystics, and healers of all traditions and cultures. The vagus nerve connects to the heart, affecting its rate and activity.

Vagotomy, or cutting the vagus nerve to the stomach, used to be standard practice during surgery for ulcers. This procedure seemed to decrease the acid in the stomach. However, such acid secretion may have been related to stress, diet, infection, and other factors.

Another gut organ that may be part of our emotional response system is the liver. In traditional Chinese medicine, the liver is considered an important element in balancing emotions. Chinese medicine uses such expressions as "rebellious liver" or "fire in the liver" to describe states often related to anger and similar hot emotions.

Certain medical conditions are often linked with emotion: ulcers with stress; irritable bowel syndrome with anxiety and stress; worsening of cramps, gas, and bloating with unconscious swallowing of air (*aerophagia*) when eating too fast, due simply to haste or to worry; and a feeling of difficulty swallowing, like a lump in the throat (*globus hystericus*), due to panic and generalized anxiety syndromes.

It can work the other way too. If your gut doesn't feel good, it can make you feel bad emotionally and in other ways. The old-fashioned expression "feeling liverish" refers to cross, foul tempers thought to be due to liver irritation, such as a bad temper caused by drinking too much alcohol and a subsequent hangover. We know that alcohol in excess affects the liver, and though the link with mood can be a centrally mediated effect on the brain, it also may come through irritation of the stomach, liver, and pancreas. We also know the phrase "quit your bellyaching" refers to a person who complains a lot, perhaps giving others a bellyache, as well.

Kids and Gut Feelings

Children may have vague and recurrent abdominal pain symptoms. As a family doctor treating children for over thirty years, I have found that such symptoms can come from a variety of causes, with emotional issues being very common. These emotional antecedents can easily be ignored or masked unless you take a holistic view of the child and family. Other causes for childhood abdominal pain may, of course, be due to serious surgical emergencies, such as appendicitis or bowel obstruction from gut tissue telescoping into itself (*intussusception*) or strangulation (*hernia* or *volvulus*). It may also be due to food allergy, lactose intolerance, constipation, and so on. But in many cases, no specific cause can be found. In that case, family stress or difficult relationships at home or in school may be major factors in childhood abdominal pain. Unless such issues are addressed, changes in diet, medications, and further testing are likely to be futile.

Our Fourth Eye

Even memories of trauma, painful experiences, injuries, insults, and emotional upset can be felt in our gut, or "viscerally retrieved." Something long past can make our gut twist in painful agony. Interesting, isn't it, how sensitive our gut is to a complex range of feelings, even memories?

You've likely heard of the "third eye" as a center of spiritual awareness and consciousness on the forehead. Perhaps the belly button, centered over our sensitive and feeling gut, is truly a "fourth eye" that helps us experience the world emotionally. It is not coincidental that many of the relaxation exercises described in this chapter center on breathing into the lower belly, using the *umbilicus*, or belly button, as a focus point.

Here is a short exercise to help you identify your gut feelings more clearly.

YOUR EMOTIONS AND YOUR GUT

Identify any or all of the following reactions to difficult emotions that are true for you. Then name the emotion causing the sensation after it, such as anger, worry, fear, love, and so on:

When you get upset, angry, fearful, frustrated, stressed out, uncertain, indecisive, or anxious, or feel other intense and difficult emotion, you notice:

A clenching, twisting feeling in your gut   Emotion _____

A burning sensation like acid dripping into your stomach   Emotion _____

Nausea   Emotion _____

Diarrhea   Emotion _____

Cramping   Emotion _____

A tightness in your belly and chest   Emotion _____

A burning sensation in your upper abdomen going into
your chest   Emotion _____

Excessive gas   Emotion _____

Pain in your rectal area   Emotion _____

Other _____   Emotion _____

Now let's check your positive emotions. Identify the reaction and name the emotion or emotions that accompany it. When you feel at peace, excited, happy, satisfied, joyful, loving, enthusiastic, or other positive emotions, you notice:

A greater appreciation and enjoyment of your meals   Emotion _____

A warm fullness in your abdomen   Emotion _____

A softening of your belly muscles   Emotion _____

A smoothness to your digestion   Emotion _____

An ease to your bowel movements   Emotion _____

Other _____   Emotion _____

If you recognized that you have a gut response to any of the above emotions, especially the negative ones, that's good! In fact, though we use the terms negative and positive, emotions and our feelings are really neither good nor bad; they are just "what is" in your current life experience. Learning to accept your feelings is good, for now you have a feedback system that will let you know if you are upset, angry, frustrated, stressed, and so on. You may note that different emotions affect your gut in very different ways.

What we might call "positive emotions" soothe us. Worry or anxiety may cause an uneasy cramping sensation or diarrhea, while anger may cause acid symptoms in the stomach or heartburn. Once you can recognize and be mindful of these early signs of emotional distress through signals your gut is giving you, you will be able to intervene. This is a process of early identification and prevention of further problems. It's an alternative to jumping right into treatment with medications such as antacids, antispasmodics, and painkillers.

Symptoms of emotional distress can sometimes be vague, like a slight burning sensation in the upper belly, bloating, heaviness, or indigestion. Try to notice new or perhaps old and familiar symptoms so that you can respond to stress or emotional upset. This is a key to helping you change unhealthy patterns of stress. The goal here is to become more mindful of how your emotions and your gut interact with each other and the world around you.

MEASURING AND MANAGING STRESS

Doctors Thomas Holmes and Richard Rahe (1967) from the University of Washington discovered that as life stressors accumulate, you are more likely to become ill. You can use the Holmes and Rahe Stress Scale to measure your current stress levels, based on recent stress factors in your life (see resources). If you score high on this scale, know that there are a broad variety of useful techniques you can use to help regulate and control your body and your stress levels.

Getting Stress Under Control

One of the best resources for addressing stress is *The Relaxation and Stress Reduction Workbook* (Davis, McKay, and Eshelman 2008). This workbook guides the reader through different techniques for managing stress and improving relaxation. These techniques include the following:

- deep breathing for general relaxation

- imagery for moving into a new mental space for relaxation

- worry/thought control for stopping intrusive, unhelpful, worrisome thoughts

- anger management for controlling anger and making it useful

- assertiveness for setting boundaries and dealing with difficult people

If you are under a lot of stress, either acutely or chronically, you may want to get a copy of this book (see resources). You can also try the following simple deep-belly breathing exercise. Practicing it regularly can help you learn to soothe your mood and your gut.

DEEP-BELLY BREATHING EXERCISE

Take the following steps to enjoy the benefits of deep-belly breathing:

1. Imagine that your lungs are in your belly.

2. As you take a deep breath, let your belly expand naturally, slowly.

3. Think "soft belly."

4. As you breathe, allow each breath to fill the lungs in your soft belly.

5. Keep the belly soft as it expands with each breath. As you exhale, squeeze the air out by pretending your belly button is going inward as if to touch your spine.

6. Ride the waves of these deep breaths for a few minutes and note how relaxed you become.

7. If worries or other thoughts distract you, return your attention to your breath.

8. Anchor your mental attention in the breath and let the warm, wonderful feeling of soft belly breathing create a calming, peaceful feeling throughout your system and throughout your day.

Anytime you notice stress or distress that affects your gut or any other part of your body, you can remind yourself of calmness by taking a few of these deep, centering breaths.

One of the reasons such a simple exercise is so effective is that as you slow and deepen your breathing, you give messages to your brain that all is safe and calm. When you are breathing fast, it is generally indicative of an alarm or stress state. By choosing to breathe slowly and deeply and moving the diaphragm muscle of the lungs deeply into the soft belly, you initiate a biofeedback loop telling you that all is well.

So try to notice the next time you feel tense and anxious. You may notice familiar gut sensations, or you may have feelings that occur elsewhere in your body. For example, you may experience muscle tension in the shoulders, shortness of breath, headache, heart palpitations, or a choking sensation. Your response is your response, neither bad nor good but information about your internal emotional state. Use it to become healthier.

By practicing relaxation and centering exercises, your body will start to get more and more comfortable with what such relaxation feels like, remembering wellness, so to speak.

The Relaxation Response

An easy exercise to learn and practice is the well-researched *relaxation response*, first used by Harvard cardiologist Herbert Benson (1975, 1984), who condensed many types of relaxation and meditation exercise into two simple steps: breathe and focus.

To elicit the relaxation response, you start with a deep breathing exercise and add a step of focusing on a certain word or phrase, which helps to quiet the mind. The word or phrase can be anything you choose, such as the word "relax," "one," "peace," or "ocean," or it can be a short prayer or phrase from your religious tradition: "The Lord is my shepherd," "God is One," and so on. The key is to make the focus word or phrase short and easy to remember and repeat mentally.

How this works is that even though you may be sitting and breathing quietly, the mind is always active and jumps from thought to thought like a monkey going from tree to tree. The anchor of breathing and the mental discipline of attending to the focus word elicit the stress-relieving relaxation response.

Try practicing the following exercise at least ten minutes once or twice daily to train your mind in how to apply it when you need it most.

PRACTICE THE RELAXATION RESPONSE

Follow these basic steps to elicit the relaxation response:

1. Sit quietly in a comfortable position.

2. Close your eyes.

3. Relax the muscles.

4. Focus on a word or phrase.

5. Breathe slowly, naturally, repeating the focus word.

6. Assume a passive attitude.

7. Continue this pattern of breathing and focus for ten to twenty minutes.

8. When distracting thoughts occur, return your attention to the focus word, and to your breathing.

If you practice this exercise regularly or daily, you can train your mind to activate a mini-relaxation vacation whenever you notice gut feelings of tension or discomfort. This could happen while you're held up at a traffic light when you are running late, before a meeting with someone who gets your gut roiling, or simply when you can't seem to shake a worrisome or negative thought or image.

Adapted from Benson and Stuart (1992)

CONCLUSION

Once you start to notice the feelings and messages your gut and other body locations are giving you, you can respond to them in new ways. You can use relaxation techniques to help you function more peacefully and calmly in all areas of your life and the world. Choose a process or technique that works best for you. With practice, you can engage, accept, and understand your feelings better. You'll feel better, your friends and family will thank you, and your gut will thank you. Your fourth eye will resonate happily as well.

PART 2

SOME THINGS YOU CAN DO FOR YOUR GUT

CHAPTER 9

COMMON CONDITIONS
THAT MAKE YOU AND
YOUR GUT SUFFER

SOME INTEGRATIVE, FUNCTIONAL,
AND HOLISTIC SOLUTIONS

This chapter takes an integrative approach to specific digestive conditions. An integrative approach includes both conventional medical and complementary therapies. Drugs are useful and even necessary for many digestive conditions, such as inflammatory bowel disease and chronic hepatitis.

While space does not allow going into great depth on all types of therapy, this chapter will help you identify some options.

As you begin your healing journey for digestive health, you need to know the evidence for and safety of various treatments. This chapter will begin with some basic principles to follow as you consider your condition and choose what treatment is right for you. Whenever in doubt, be sure to meet with your health care provider, be it a physician, nurse practitioner, naturopathic doctor, nutritionist, or complementary medicine expert. Come prepared to discuss your thoughts, concerns, and knowledge. Bring any printed information you feel is relevant. You need to take full advantage of the broadest possible range of options to enhance your GI health and, along with it, reduce your risk of health problems in other body systems.

MAKING SOUND HEALTH DECISIONS FOR YOURSELF AND YOUR FAMILY

In addressing any health concern, consider the following dimensions of your condition: acuteness, severity, and chronicity of the problem and evidence for different treatments.

Acuteness

Is it a brief, likely self-limited condition—that is, something that is likely to go away by itself, such as stomach flu? If you have never had this condition before, do you know from friends or family that it is likely to be brief and, even if uncomfortable, something you can manage with simple measures and without medical attention? If you don't know, assume it could be more serious and get checked out professionally.

Severity

Is it potentially and significantly hazardous to your health, either short term—for example, severe abdominal pain (appendicitis, perforated ulcer)—or long term (inflammatory bowel disease, hepatitis, pancreatitis)? Is there an immediate risk to you of major medical complications, such as bleeding, dehydration, or infection?

Chronicity

If it is a condition that is long lasting, what are the risks and benefits of various therapies that are available? What are their costs? How would they affect your lifestyle, and what changes in lifestyle are you willing to make? Have you considered all your possible options?

Evidence

Making wise choices for your and your family's health requires a basic knowledge of the evidence for certain treatments. The term *evidence* or *evidence-based* in medical science refers to the level of scientific support for a treatment based on quality clinical trials. These are usually randomized, controlled, double-blind trials (RCDBTs) or meta-analyses in which the results of multiple studies are pooled. In double-blind trials, neither the researcher nor the subject knows if the subject is receiving an active or a placebo treatment. This experimental method is useful for drug studies but less helpful in integrative approaches, which use multiple interventions, nutritional studies, and hands-on methods like massage, acupuncture, or manipulative therapies, where "blinding" the subject and researcher is very difficult or impossible. The RCDBT is also not highly suitable for examining the kind of complex lifestyle changes that can be so vital to your overall health. Scientific support for traditional cultural and home therapies, nutritional and lifestyle approaches, mind-body methods, supplements, and botanicals is likewise in a state of evolution. The evidence for some of these types of therapies can be based on inferences drawn from centuries-old traditional practices; complex theory and whole science approaches, which test how such multiple therapies are used in the real world; expert consensus; best-case series; and even individualized "N of 1" studies, in which individuals serve as their own control group.

While many standard medical and surgical therapies are supported by well-done research, you may be surprised to know that less than 30 percent meet the highest standards of evidence for safety and effectiveness (RCDBTs and meta-analyses). We often see medications, proven and reported to be useful through standard scientific methods and publications, taken off the market for safety reasons. Today's standard treatment may be replaced by tomorrow's new method. A good rule of thumb is "Don't be the first to adopt a new treatment nor the last to abandon the old one." Be aware that medical science is in constant flux. So final evidence is often in flux, uncertain, or absent.

Be aware that what passes for evidence, particularly in the popular press and on the Internet, is often promotional material, testimonials from doctors and consumers, promises of cost-savings, and claims of safety and efficacy that exceed scientific fact. Infomercials are designed to sell you products that you may not need and may be just a waste of time and money. Even worse, they may be unsafe.

Safety matters. It is usually more important than the potential or marginal benefit from a new drug, a new surgical technique, or the latest supplement to hit a multi-level marketing scheme. So how do you choose among the variety of options available for many conditions? Of overarching concern is the balance between safety and effectiveness.

Ask yourself the following questions:

1. Is the treatment for a certain condition proven to be both safe and effective (e.g., antibiotics for diverticulitis, chemotherapy/antiviral therapy for hepatitis B)? If so, use this treatment.

2. Is the treatment safe but you are unsure whether it is effective (e.g., peppermint oil or relaxation therapies for irritable bowel syndrome)? If so, consider using this therapy if treatment 1 does not work, has intolerable side effects, or is too costly, or there is no proven effective therapy for the condition.

3. Is the treatment unsafe, or potentially so, and only possibly effective (e.g., an unknown Chinese herbal mixture for ulcers without the advice of an expert in Chinese medicine)? If so, take this therapy only if nothing else works and you are willing to take a risk on safety.

4. Is the treatment both unsafe and ineffective (e.g., liver toxic herbs, like chaparral, for cancer)? If so, do not take this therapy.

So that is the consideration on choosing a therapy. While you might presume that medications on the market are safe and proven, this is not always the case (see chapter 10). Nor is it true that so-called natural therapies are always safe. The level of evidence for some of these complementary therapies is also less than robust in some cases, though their toxicity or potential for harm is generally less than that of many prescription medications.

The choices you will have to make, with the advice of your physician as needed, are outlined in figures 4 and 5:

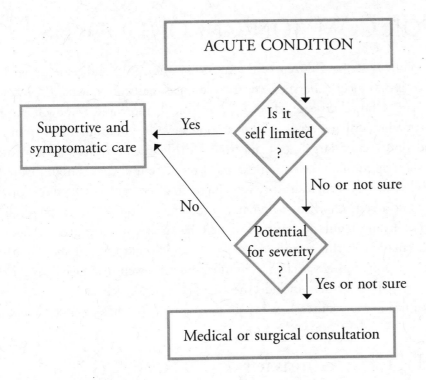

FIGURE 4: ACUTE CONDITION

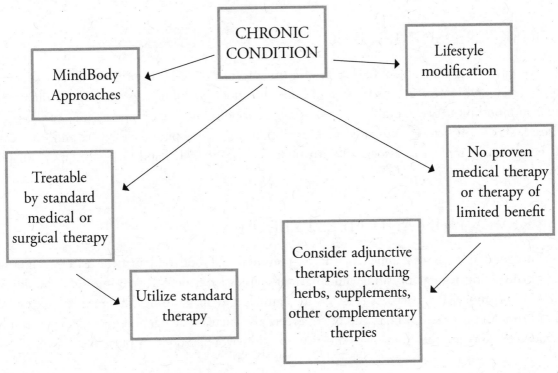

FIGURE 5: CHRONIC CONDITION

REMEDIES FOR COMMON GI CONDITIONS

The text and tables that follow describe a dozen of the most common GI conditions (gingivitis, heartburn and reflux, gastritis and ulcers, diarrhea, constipation, gas, gallstones, hepatitis, irritable bowel syndrome, inflammatory bowel disease, diverticulosis, and hemorrhoids) and offer some perspective on selecting remedies. All materials in this section have been summarized from the latest medical recommendations, based largely on data from UpToDate and other recent medical literature. UpToDate is a subscription-based electronic clinical resource tool that is highly popular among physicians, medical students, and residents, for whom it often replaces textbooks. It is extremely useful in the clinical setting when facing new problems or those not responding as expected. All recommendations are regularly updated as new research comes in and changes in therapies occur. Other information in this section relies on scientific references, medical research materials, books, websites, and other sources as cited. A number of useful websites, such as WebMD, are free and available to the public. Others include the Mayo Clinic, which can also help you access the information you need (see resources). When in doubt, talk to a health professional.

More Than Halitosis: Gingivitis

Gingivitis is an inflammation of the gums characterized by redness, swelling, and a tendency to bleed.

RISK AND SIGNIFICANCE

We have long known about the risk of gum infections to oral health, causing problems like tooth decay and tooth loss, abscesses, and bone infection. New findings show that inflammation is a common link between oral and many systemic conditions. Conditions such as cardiovascular disease, stroke, diabetes, rheumatoid arthritis, renal disease, respiratory disease, and even cancer all have been described as associated with poor oral health (Michaud et al. 2008; Scannapieco, Bush, and Paju 2003).

PREVENTION AND LIFESTYLE

The good news is that much of this is preventable. Good oral hygiene is a commonsense matter involving regular brushing, flossing, and professional dental cleaning. You should avoid smoking or smokeless tobacco as these create significant damage to healthy gums. High-glycemic foods, simple sugars, soft drinks, and other sweets also increase dental and gum damage. You have already seen lots of other reasons to substitute healthier SuperFoods in place of these.

STANDARD THERAPY

When infections get advanced, antibiotics orally and systemically are used. Sometimes gum surgery is necessary.

INTEGRATIVE APPROACHES

To protect the gums and the rest of your system as well, you can use a variety of botanical and nutritional supplements that are listed in the table that follows. These have a number of mechanisms. For example, vitamin C (Woolfe et al. 1984; Vaananen et al. 1993), flavonoids, and grapeseed extract are antioxidants that reduce free radical damage and thereby decrease inflammation. Coenzyme Q10 is another antioxidant but also is an important contributor to energy metabolism in the *mitochondria*, the individual body cell's "power packs." You can chew a CoQ10 gelcap before bedtime after flossing and brushing to allow it to be in direct contact with the gums (Wilkinson, Arnold, and Folkers 1976; Nakamura et al. 1973). A number of rinses such as aloe, folic acid, and tea tree oil help keep the gums cleansed. They are also antibacterial. Vitamins like folic acid (Pack 1984), vitamin D, and minerals such as zinc keep the local immune system functioning better.

While you likely won't want to try all of these together, pick a mouth rinse plus supplements that you suspect you might be lacking, depending on your diet and lifestyle habits and specific nutrient testing.

Condition	Lifestyle Options	Conventional Medical/Surgical Approaches	Botanical and Nutritional Supplements	Other Integrative, Functional, Holistic Solutions
Gingivitis	• Regular brushing (consider electric toothbrush) • Flossing twice daily • Biannual dental cleaning • Avoiding simple sugars, soft drinks, candies • Avoiding tobacco products in any form	• Chlorhexidine 0.12 percent mouthwash • Antibiotics (metronidazole, amoxicillin-clavulanate, ampicillin-sulbactam, or clindamycin) • Dental fluoridation • Surgical debridement and repair	• Aloe vera juice (topically, swish and rinse three times daily) • Chamomile (strong tea of two to three teabags in a cup as mouthwash, two to three times daily) • Coenzyme Q10 (50 to 100 mg daily) • Folic acid rinse (one teaspoon 0.1 percent solution twice daily) • Grapeseed extract (take one 25 to 100 mg capsule one to three times daily) • Hyaluronic acid (topically twice daily) • Tea tree oil (five to six drops in water as mouthwash, two to three times daily) • Vitamin C (300 mg daily) plus flavonoid supplementation for those with diets low in fruits and vegetables • Vitamin D (400 to 2000 IU daily) • Zinc (15 to 30 mg daily)	• Swishing with green or black tea two to three times daily • Eating a small box of raisins daily • Toothpaste with bloodroot (may include sage oil, peppermint oil, menthol, chamomile, clove, caraway oil)

Up the Down Staircase: Heartburn and Reflux

Gastroesophageal reflux disease (GERD) is a condition in which a burning sensation (heartburn) is felt in the upper abdomen, the middle of the chest, and the throat due to abnormal passage (reflux) of stomach acid and contents into the esophagus. This is usually due to decreased tone of the lower esophageal sphincter, a hiatal hernia (a bulge of a portion of the stomach through the diaphragm where the esophagus normally passes), or increased intra-abdominal pressure.

RISK AND SIGNIFICANCE

Affecting up to 8 percent of the population, GERD is a cause of significant symptoms for many with GI-related conditions. The discomfort associated with heartburn and reflux can be mistaken for a heart attack, a gallbladder attack, or heart or lung problems. If inadequately managed, GERD can cause chronic hoarseness, pain or difficulty in swallowing, worsening of asthma, and increased risk for pneumonia (Laheij 2004), as well as increased risk of esophageal cancer (Shaheen and Ransohoff 2002).

PREVENTION AND LIFESTYLE

Lifestyle issues are important in GERD. Maintaining a normal weight and regular stool habits is important. This is because being overweight, constipation, or even tight-fitting garments increase the intra-abdominal pressure and risk of hiatal hernia that worsen GERD. Smoking, caffeine, alcohol, and certain other foods aggravate GERD and should be avoided. Smoking also lessens saliva secretion, reducing your ability to neutralize acid with the basic (high pH) saliva. You generally will recognize culprit foods, but common ones are spicy foods, peppermint, chocolate, and fatty foods. Don't go to bed less than two hours after eating if you have this condition, as a full stomach is prone to release contents into the esophagus. Eat small meals to prevent over-distending the stomach and increasing pressure on the lower esophageal sphincter. For chronic nighttime symptoms, elevating the head of the bed six to eight inches on blocks will help gravity to move food downstream.

STANDARD THERAPY

The approach to GERD depends on many factors, including severity, chronicity, associated symptoms, and complications. Typically for occasional heartburn, an over-the-counter antacid or H2 blocker is adequate. If symptoms progress and persist, proton pump inhibitors (PPIs) may be started, and infection with *H. pylori* is treated if present. Because of the risk of these medications, a step-up and step-down therapy approach is often used (see chapter 10).

Surveillance with endoscopy (EGD) is sometimes indicated in cases that fail to respond and also to monitor for the presence of Barrett's esophagus, a condition that can be preliminary to cancer. Surgery is occasionally done to repair a large hiatal hernia, which can cause GERD unresponsive to other measures.

INTEGRATIVE APPROACHES

In addition to commonsense lifestyle and preventive measures, some herbal supplements can be helpful. Deglycyrrhizinated licorice (DGL) is a product that soothes and coats the esophagus and stomach, acts as an antacid, and may combat *H. pylori* infection. Other demulcents and healing agents like slippery elm, aloe vera juice, and rice bran oil may be useful in acute or chronic conditions. If these do not work, you should not hesitate to take prescription medications. Even chewing gum for milder cases of GERD can be useful as the saliva neutralizes the acid in the esophagus. Mindful eating, chewing, and swallowing help digest food better, mix in more saliva, and give your stomach acids time to work. All of these can reduce GERD.

Condition	Lifestyle Options	Conventional Medical/Surgical Approaches	Botanical and Nutritional Supplements	Other Integrative, Functional, Holistic Solutions
Esophagitis and gastroesophageal reflux disease	• Eating smaller meals • Avoiding eating two to three hours before going to bed • Elevating head of bed by six to eight inches to reduce reflux • Avoiding offending foods and beverages (caffeine, alcohol, chocolate, mint, spicy foods, onions, peppers, fatty foods) • Quitting smoking • Losing weight • Avoiding tight-fitting garments	• Antacid therapy: Maalox, Mylanta, Gaviscon, TUMS • H2 blockers: ranitidine/Zantac (150 mg twice daily or 300 mg at bedtime, maintenance therapy 150 mg at bedtime); famotidine/Pepcid (20 mg twice daily, 40 mg at bedtime, maintenance 20 mg at bedtime); cimetidine/Tagamet (400 mg twice daily or 800 mg at bedtime, maintenance 400 mg at bedtime); nizatidine/Axid (150 mg twice daily, 300 mg at bedtime, maintenance 150 mg at bedtime) • Proton pump inhibitors: omperazole/Prilosec (20 to 40 mg daily); pantoprazole/Protonix (15 to 30 mg daily); esomeprazole/Nexium (20 to 80 mg daily); rabeparazole/Aciphex (20 mg daily) • Testing for *H. pylori* and treating in acute cases with proton pump inhibitors and antibiotics (not for chronic GERD symptoms). Dosages of PPIs are adjusted when used with antibiotics. • Esophageal acid monitoring (pH monitor) • Endoscopy of esophagus and stomach (EGD) • Dilation of narrowed esophagus • Surgical repair of hiatal hernia	• Aloe vera juice (half cup three times daily) • DGL (two to four tablets 380 mg before meals) • Rice bran oil (150 mg three times a day for a month) • Slippery elm (two tablespoons mixed in water after meals and at bedtime)	• Stress management and relaxation techniques • Mindful eating with slower chewing, swallowing • Eating bananas • Drinking eight to ten glasses of water daily • Chewing gum

Acid Trip: Gastritis and Ulcers

Gastritis is an acute or chronic inflammation of the lining of the stomach. A peptic ulcer is a break in the lining of the stomach. Both conditions are caused by an imbalance of the mucous membrane factors in the stomach and the strong acid that is secreted there. Infection with *H. pylori,* autoimmune and hypersensitivity reactions, medications, tobacco, alcohol, and other lifestyle factors may damage the protective factors in the stomach and cause gastritis or ulcers.

RISK AND SIGNIFICANCE

Untreated, ulcers and gastritis cause chronic pain, bleeding, or scarring. These conditions represent a spectrum of disease starting with irritation and leading to frank ulceration.

Gastritis is almost always associated with *H. pylori* infection, though it can also be caused by medications and autoimmune and hypersensitivity reactions. *Gastropathy* is a noninflammatory condition secondary to irritants, such as bile reflux, alcohol, NSAIDs, or aspirin. Gastropathy can also be due to stress, chronic congestion, or decreased blood flow to the stomach. Biopsy of the lining of the stomach can distinguish between gastritis (acute or chronic) and gastropathy. *Atrophic gastritis* is due to loss of gastric mucosa and acid secretion and can cause multiple risks of nutrient deficiency—for example, vitamin B_{12} deficiency and subsequent anemia and gastric cancer. Familial and genetic factors play a role in risk as well.

Peptic ulcers are so named to distinguish them from other kinds of ulcers like diabetic ulcers or *decubitus* (bedsore) ulcers. They are typically located in the duodenum. This kind of ulcer is commonly associated with *H. pylori* infection as well and so requires eradication of this organism, if present, for successful treatment. However, peptic ulcers may be recurrent in a high percentage of cases, despite therapy. So-called gastric ulcers or giant ulcers occurring in the body of the stomach may be malignant and need to be biopsied.

PREVENTION AND LIFESTYLE

Diet approaches have not really been shown to significantly affect gastritis and ulcers. It used to be thought that dairy products like milk relieved symptoms of ulcers, but it was later found that milk products actually increased acid secretion. Fermented milk products seem to be more helpful, however.

Removing irritant agents is definitely helpful. I recommend stress-management measures for gastritis and ulcers; the medical literature has long discussed this but focuses less on it now, perhaps because of the causative factor of infection now found in these diseases (Bhatia and Tandon 2005; Levenstein et al. 1999). Nonetheless, lowering levels of stress can reduce adrenaline and cortisone secretions, both of which can affect blood flow and the protective mechanisms in the stomach, and can also improve other conditions. Furthermore, people in high-stress situations, such as war and natural disasters, are seen to have higher risk of peptic ulcers. Regular exercise and adequate sleep can also relieve stress and reduce risk of these conditions.

STANDARD THERAPY

General principles for both gastritis and ulcers are to provide suppression of acid secretion, *H. pylori* eradication, and removal of offending causes. Some patients are at higher risk for recurrence (smokers, chronic NSAID users) and likely will require maintenance therapy. Medications have improved in terms of potency and effectiveness, and for most people, medications are the first line of treatment.

Various protocols have emerged over the years, but most practically speaking, at the onset of symptoms, I recommend taking either an H2 blocker or a proton pump inhibitor, based on severity and risk factors. If no relief after a couple weeks, I check for *H. pylori* and continue with the same or a doubled dose of medication for up to a month. If no relief, I refer for endoscopy.

Surgery, which used to be a mainstay of ulcer treatment in the past generation (the vagotomy and pyloroplasty procedure), is now rarely necessary except in the case of bleeding untreatable by endoscopy or medications. It is also used to reduce blockage from scarring in the duodenum, which is seen less often now that more effective treatments are available.

INTEGRATIVE APPROACHES

Given the effectiveness of medications in gastritis and ulcers, what is the role of complementary approaches? First, recall that there is a high recurrence rate, despite optimal medical management. Second, long-term acid suppressive therapy is not without risks.

DGL, mastic gum, aloe, even cabbage juice, along with vitamins, minerals, and essential fatty acids, can help heal ulcers, boost immunity, and suppress *H. pylori* (Brogden, Speight, and Avery 1974; Huwez et al. 1998; Cheney 1949; Kockar, Ozturk, and Bavbek 2001; Kamiji and de Oliveira 2005). Any of these approaches can be tried if you do not respond to conventional medications, have intolerable side effects or allergic reactions, cannot afford medicine, or are interested in reducing the risks of recurrence. Remember to use probiotic support if you have been treated with antibiotics for *H. pylori* (Sullivan and Nord 2005).

Condition	Lifestyle Options	Conventional Medical/Surgical Approaches	Botanical and Nutritional Supplements	Other Integrative, Functional, Holistic Solutions
Gastritis and ulcers	• Avoiding milk products except yogurt/kefir • Eating breakfast and regular meals • Avoiding large meals • Avoiding caffeine, tobacco, offending drugs (aspirin, steroids, and NSAIDs, like ibuprofen, naproxen) • Getting regular exercise • Getting adequate sleep	• Antacid therapy: Maalox, Mylanta, Gaviscon, TUMS • H2 blockers: ranitidine/Zantac (150 mg twice daily or 300 mg at bedtime, maintenance therapy 150 mg at bedtime); famotidine/Pepcid (20 mg twice daily, 40 mg at bedtime, maintenance 20 mg at bedtime); cimetidine/Tagamet (400 mg twice daily or 800 mg at bedtime, maintenance 400 mg at bedtime); nizatidine/Axid (150 mg twice daily, 300 mg at bedtime, maintenance 150 mg at bedtime) • Proton pump inhibitors: omperazole/Prilosec (20 to 40 mg daily); pantoprazole/Protonix (15 to 30 mg daily); esomeprazole/Nexium (20 to 80 mg daily); rabeparazole/Aciphex (20 mg daily) • Testing for *H. pylori* and treating when positive with PPI and antibiotics. Dosages of PPIs are adjusted when used with antibiotics. • Endoscopy of esophagus and stomach (EGD) • Surgery for bleeding, scarring	• DGL (two to four tablets 380 mg before meals for acute ulcer or gastritis, one to two tablets for chronic condition) • Mastic gum (500 mg three times daily) • Slippery elm (500 mg three times daily) • Aloe vera juice (half cup three times daily) • Cabbage juice (one glass twice daily) • Chamomile tea (three cups daily) • Turmeric (600 mg five times daily) • Vitamin C (1200 to 5000 mg a day to suppress *H. pylori* (no more than 500 mg a dose, up to four weeks total) • Zinc (30 to 50 mg daily as arginate or hydrate form for three to six weeks, supplement with at least 1 to 2 mg copper daily) • Glutamine (1600 to 3000 mg in three to four divided doses for four weeks) • Fish oil and black currant oil (1 g of each daily for eight weeks for suppression of *H. pylori*)	• Stress reduction measures • Whole grains • Fiber • Pumpkin seeds (zinc source) • Probiotics (5 to 20 billion units twice a day during and following antibiotic use for at least two weeks)

Too Fast: Diarrhea

Diarrhea is the passage of fluids or unformed stools in increased frequency compared to normal bowel movements.

RISK AND SIGNIFICANCE

Diarrhea is not a disease; it is a symptom. Most commonly it is due to infectious conditions, such as viruses, bacteria, or other pathogenic organisms. By and large, diarrhea is a self-limited condition. If it is chronic, it can be from conditions such as irritable bowel syndrome or inflammatory bowel disease, which require different approaches, as noted further in this chapter.

Treatment is generally supportive and aimed at avoiding dehydration and relieving symptoms. Diarrhea is a serious cause of death in developing countries, especially among children, but is less likely to be life-threatening elsewhere. Diarrhea accompanied by fever or bloody diarrhea is more likely to be from an invasive infection and may require antibiotics.

PREVENTION AND LIFESTYLE

Wash your hands regularly if you have diarrhea to prevent spreading infection to others. To prevent traveler's diarrhea, be sure to wash fruits and vegetables thoroughly and use bottled or boiled water. These measures are particularly important when traveling in developing countries. Take probiotics if you are taking antibiotics for diarrhea.

STANDARD THERAPY

Acute diarrhea (less than fourteen days in duration) is treated supportively by maintaining hydration. In milder cases, soups, broths, clear liquids, diluted juices, water, and sweat replacement fluids like Gatorade may be adequate. Dietary modification is also recommended. If you do not have bloody diarrhea or fever, symptomatic support may be given with loperamide or diphenoxylate to slow stools and reduce cramping.

You will need medical evaluation if you have such voluminous stools that you are getting dehydrated (signaled by poor skin tone, dry mouth, faintness, weakness). Other danger signs suggesting that you require medical attention are fever (≥101.3° F, ≥38.5° C), bloody diarrhea, six stools or more in twenty-four hours, severe abdominal pain, recent hospitalization or antibiotic use, age over seventy or under two years, or if you are immunocompromised.

Traveler's diarrhea needs a special approach if persistent and often, depending on where you acquired it. This condition may require antibiotics for bacteria like *E. coli* or for parasites like *Giardia* or amoebas.

Persistent diarrhea, lasting more than two weeks, and certainly chronic diarrhea, lasting longer than four weeks, will require medical consultation.

INTEGRATIVE APPROACHES

Perhaps the most useful approach is to remember to use probiotics during acute diarrhea (to shorten the course) and afterwards (to help reestablish normal gut bacteria) (Saavedra 2000, 2002). This is especially the case if you are taking antibiotics for any reason. Avoid magnesium and vitamin C during diarrhea as they can worsen the condition. Review your medications for any that aggravate or cause diarrhea. Many herbs and supplements as listed in the table have been traditionally used to treat diarrhea. Various berries have long been used for diarrhea. Ginger (particularly useful if you have nausea), glutamine, and slippery elm all help heal the gut and quell inflammation. Bulk-forming agents are also helpful in most cases. Be aware that the bismuth in Pepto-Bismol may turn stools black.

Condition	Lifestyle Options	Conventional Medical/Surgical Approaches	Botanical and Nutritional Supplements	Other Integrative, Functional, Holistic Solutions
Diarrhea	• Pushing fluids • BRAT diet (bananas, rice, applesauce, toast) • Eating yogurt • Reviewing medications as causative factors, e.g., antacids, antibiotics • Handwashing to prevent transmission of infection	• World Health Organization's rehydration formula: 3.5 g sodium chloride, 2.9 g trisodium citrate or 2.5 g sodium bicarbonate, 1.5 g potassium chloride, 20 g glucose or 40 g sucrose (prepare at home using one-half teaspoon of salt, one-half teaspoon of baking soda, four tablespoons of sugar, one liter of water) • Anti-motility agents: loperamide/Imodium (4 mg to start and 2 mg after each unformed stool to a maximum of 16 mg daily no more than two days); diphenoxylate/Lomotil (4 mg up to four times daily for no more than two days). Caution: use either sparingly and avoid if fever or bloody diarrhea. • Likely infectious diarrheas will need physician consultation (may need lab studies of stool). • Prescriptions may include antibiotics (ciprofloxacin, levofloxacin, trimethoprim/sulfamethoxazole, doxycycline, azithromycin, erythromycin, vancomycin); antiparasitics (metronidazole).	• Bilberry: capsules (240 to 600 mg per day) or tincture (1 to 2 ml two times per day); fruit (20 to 60 g); juice (one-half cup two to three times daily) • Ginger (500 mg twice daily or one to two cups ginger tea daily) • Glutamine (1000 to 3000 mg three times daily) • Red raspberry, blackberry, or blueberry leaf tea (one to two teaspoons dried leaves in cup of boiling water) or capsule form (5 to 10 mg daily) • Slippery elm tea (three cups daily, or 500 mg capsule daily for three days) • Zinc can improve response to triple antibiotic therapy for *H. pylori*. • Avoid magnesium and vitamin C during diarrhea.	• Probiotics to reestablish bacterial balance (two to six capsules *Lactobacillus* and *Bifidobacteria* at least 4 billion units daily); consider especially in antibiotic-induced diarrhea. • Bulk-forming agents (Kaopectate, Metamucil, psyllium) • Anti-inflammatory agents (Pepto-Bismol) • Use lactase (Lactaid) if dairy/lactose intolerance suspected (chronic diarrhea).

Too Slow: Constipation

Constipation is a decrease in frequency of a person's normal stool habit, possibly accompanied by difficulty in passage of hard, dry, or large stools.

RISK AND SIGNIFICANCE

Constipation is the most common digestive complaint in the general population (Stewart et al. 1999). Like diarrhea, constipation is not really a disease but is a result of an imbalance in bowel motility, stool bulk, fluids in the stool, and dietary factors. At times psychological factors, such as anxiety about what is a normal frequency for bowel movements, come into play.

Constipation can also be a symptom. Failure to pass stool regularly can signify a serious medical condition, such as obstruction of the bowel, diseases such as hypothyroidism, diabetes, and neurological conditions. Many medications can be constipating. Inactivity and confinement to bed or hospitalization can also contribute to constipation.

Generally speaking, constipation can occur with either normal or slow transit time in the colon, as well as loss of coordination of pelvic floor muscles and the anorectal muscles (*dyssynergy*).

PREVENTION AND LIFESTYLE

Regular exercise, adequate intake of fluids, and a high-fiber diet are sufficient for most people to prevent constipation. Avoid drugs such as opioids that are constipating, or if you must take them, use in combination with increased fluid, fiber, and/or stool softeners. A bowel-habit diary is useful to document frequency of stools and their consistency, as it helps make a more objective assessment of bowel patterns.

STANDARD THERAPY

Standard therapy involves a full evaluation to eliminate treatable or secondary causes of chronic constipation, along with patient education, dietary modification, and judicious use of laxatives and enemas. One of the most common and reversible causes of constipation is the use of drugs. These include pain medicines, particularly opioids, antihypertensives (for example, calcium channel blockers), medications such as antispasmodics, antihistamines, antidepressants, and antipsychotics, iron supplements, and aluminum-containing antacids (like Maalox and sucralfate).

Once serious or reversible causes of constipation have been excluded, a goal of treatment is to prevent overreliance on laxatives and other measures like enemas. This requires changing expectations about normal bowel habits, altering diet, exercise, and fluid intake, and encouragement that "normal" bowel habits comprise a spectrum of personal habits and frequency of stools.

INTEGRATIVE APPROACHES

Integrative approaches include many of the conventional measures and utilize an expanded list of botanical and nutritional supplements. Biofeedback can be useful, particularly in cases where dyssynergy occurs (Heymen et al. 2003). Soluble fiber is essential and probiotics, while generally used for diarrhea, are worth a try in constipation. Regular physical activity is extremely important (Peters et al. 2001).

Condition	Lifestyle Options	Conventional Medical/Surgical Approaches	Botanical and Nutritional Supplements	Other Integrative, Functional, Holistic Solutions
Constipation	• Drinking fluids (ten to twelve glasses daily) • Consuming fiber (30 g daily) from fruits, vegetables, legumes, whole grains in diet • Considering lactose intolerance • Exercising regularly • Reviewing medications that may be constipating • Keeping a weeklong bowel habit diary	• Excluding significant medical or surgical conditions through careful history, physical examinations, and if needed X-rays, endoscopy, or other tests • Education about the condition: normal vs. abnormal stool patterns, stooling after meals; avoiding excessive use of laxatives; increasing fiber and fluids, physical activity • Dietary changes: generally adding fiber and other bulk-forming agents, such as psyllium, methylcellulose, or calcium polycarbophil, though these may not be as useful in slow-transit-time type constipation • Careful use of laxatives and enemas when needed: docusate, milk of magnesia, magnesium citrate, polyethylene glycol, sorbitol, lactulose, bisacodyl, senna; saline or mineral oil enemas • Manual disimpaction • Surgery (rarely) primarily for neurological causes	• Aloe vera juice (half cup up to three times daily or 40 to 170 mg dehydrated juice in capsule to create soft stool; short-term use only, less than one week) • Cascara (250 mg two to three times daily; short term use only, less than one week) • Magnesium (350 to 500 mg a day in chelated form) • Milk of magnesia (one to two tablespoons daily) • Senna (tea with one-half teaspoon of senna in cup of water once or twice daily; may double if needed to obtain soft stool) • Vitamin C (500 to 2000 mg a day or more to achieve soft stools)	• Biofeedback in chronic cases, especially in children and in cases with dyssynergy as cause of constipation • Maintaining regular probiotic intake (*Bifidobacteria* two to three times daily) • Soluble fiber such as psyllium, ground flaxseed (one to three tablespoons daily) • Wheat or corn bran (one tablespoon daily)

Natural Gas or Unnatural? Flatulence and Belching

Flatulence is a product of digestion and intestinal bacteria composed of oxygen, nitrogen, hydrogen, carbon dioxide, methane, and hydrogen sulfide. The term *flatus* comes from the Latin for "blowing." The average person expels 400 to 1200 cubic centimeters of gas daily, in a dozen to as many as a hundred releases over the course of the day. Men and women pass similar amounts. Excessive gas in the upper GI tract may also result in belching, burping, and bloating, especially from swallowing air during eating and drinking and due to anxiety.

RISK AND SIGNIFICANCE

Flatulence is a byproduct of normal digestion. Though it may be at times socially embarrassing, it is not a disease. Those with excessive gas may also note bloating and abdominal discomfort (Lasser, Bond, and Levitt 1975).

Excessive gas commonly results from swallowing air during eating, malabsorption of certain foods, or the tendency for certain foods or carbonated beverages to produce extra gas. Other causes include irritable bowel syndrome, bowel obstruction (which reduces reabsorption of gas), decreased bowel motility in conditions like diabetes, and bacterial overgrowth or infection. Psychiatric illnesses like anxiety that cause hyperventilation and gulping air contribute to excess gas. Even changes in atmospheric pressure, such as going up in an airplane, allow gas in the bowel to expand and encourage flatulence.

PREVENTION AND LIFESTYLE

Preventing the gas problem is often a matter of trial and error. You can start by noticing the kinds of foods and beverages that increase your tendency to burp (*eructate*) or pass gas. A food diary is helpful in this approach.

In some cases, extra gas is due to food allergy, malabsorption of carbohydrates or other foods, or lack of specific enzymes like lactase for dairy or pancreatic enzymes for protein, carbohydrates, or fats. Keeping a careful diary can help to identify these problems. You can also pay attention to any behavioral or mood problems that may be contributing to excessive gas and address these through psychotherapy, medications, and relaxation exercises.

STANDARD THERAPY

Conventional therapy examines possible problems, such as gallbladder disease, food allergy or intolerance, infections, or surgical issues requiring immediate attention. Once this evaluation has been done, dietary modifications, appropriate psychological treatments, such as treatment of anxiety for *aerophagia* (air swallowing) (Chitkara et al. 2005), and some medications, like simethicone, remain the mainstay of treatment.

INTEGRATIVE APPROACHES

A number of traditional herbs and supplements are useful for reducing gas. Mindful eating to reduce swallowing of air is worth considering. Many of the issues that have been discussed in this book related to food allergy and intolerances are relevant to reducing excess gas. If changes in diet and lifestyle are ineffective, you may want to consider products like Beano (Ganiats et al. 1994), Mylicon, Lactaid, or activated charcoal (Potter, Ellis, and Levitt 1985). A trial of digestive enzymes may be worthwhile if you suspect insufficiency of stomach, liver, or pancreatic digestive secretions. These might include hydrochloric acid (betaine hydrochloride), bile salts, bromelain, papain, or pancreatic enzymes. I recommend a consultation with a nutritionist or holistic practitioner familiar with these supplements.

Condition	Lifestyle Options	Conventional Medical/ Surgical Approaches	Botanical and Nutritional Supplements	Other Integrative, Functional, Holistic Solutions
Gas (belching and flatulence)	• Addressing food allergy, intolerance, lactose intolerance where present • Avoiding offending foods which may be one or more of the following: apples, apricots, bananas, beans, broccoli, brussels sprouts, cabbage, cauliflower, corn, dairy, high-fiber cereals, lentils, oats, onions, peaches, pears, prunes, raisins, wheat • Chewing more slowly • Soaking beans overnight before cooking • Avoiding carbonated beverages	• Determine if the complaint is one of excess passing of gas, belching, or simply a subjective feeling of bloating For belching: • Reducing aerophagia through education • Discontinuation of gum chewing, smoking, drinking carbonated beverages, and gulping food and liquids For intestinal gas: • Avoiding lactose • Avoiding fructose • Avoiding sorbitol (may be contained in dietetic foods and chewing gum) • Avoiding foods known to promote gaseousness (legumes and cruciferous vegetables) • Breath testing for bacterial overgrowth if suspected	• Anise (make tea from one teaspoon crushed seeds and take several times daily) • Caraway (eat half a teaspoon of seeds chewed after a meal, or make a tea with one to two teaspoons of crushed seeds and hot water and take as needed) • Chlorophyll (liquid or tablets two to three times daily with meals) • Peppermint (one tablespoon of leaves with a cup of boiling water to make tea three times daily, or if heartburn occurs, take enteric-coated capsules three times daily) • Dill (one teaspoon ground seeds in a cup of hot water to make tea). Drink as needed. For stronger effect, use one teaspoon dill oil in four cups of water and sip as needed. • Fennel (eat one-half teaspoon seeds after meals, or make tea with one-half teaspoon powdered seeds and drink two to three times daily, or take thirty to sixty drops tincture of seeds three times daily) • Ginger (1 g, about the size of your little finger, cut up in hot water and steeped for tea to sip three times daily) • Hydrochloric acid (10 mg capsule with meals, increase by one capsule until burning is noted in the stomach, maximum five capsules per meal); useful especially for upper abdominal gas but may help with overall digestion and flatus if stomach acid is low	• Addressing anxiety issues that may be creating air-swallowing behaviors • Mindful eating • Beano (alpha-D-galactosidase inhibitor) • Charcoal tablets (one to two before meals); caution: may interfere with absorption of medications and supplements • Simethicone (80 mg three times daily) • Trial of digestive enzymes: bromelain, papaya, or pancreatic enzyme (one to two capsules with meals)

Bag of Stones: Gallstones

Gallstones are caused by the crystallization of bile high in cholesterol concentration and result from inflammation of the gallbladder often related to a high-fat diet. Gallstones can create colicky pain in the right upper part of the abdomen. They are often associated with abdominal bloating, dyspepsia, heartburn, fat intolerance, nausea, and vomiting. However, not all cases of gallstones give such symptoms.

RISK AND SIGNIFICANCE

Gallstones may be silent and create no symptoms, cause pain and inflammation requiring medications or surgery, or block the bile duct causing jaundice and liver damage. When gallstones are identified by clinical suspicion and confirmed by ultrasound imaging, the approach should be personalized according to the patient's other medical conditions and degree of symptoms. For example, diabetics with nonsymptomatic stones ought to consider surgery because of the risk of complications like gangrene if they get an attack. An eighty-year-old who has heart disease and gallstones with minimal symptoms might best be advised to do watchful waiting.

PREVENTION AND LIFESTYLE

The best way to manage gallstones is to prevent them from happening in the first place. This can be achieved through a low-fat and high-fiber diet, regular exercise (Misciagna et al. 1999), and maintaining a healthy weight. Stasis of bile in the gallbladder can promote gallstones. This can be worsened by estrogens during pregnancy, in birth control pills, and in hormonal treatements for menopausal symptoms (Grodstein et al. 1994; Simon et al. 1998). Women around age forty, especially if overweight, are at highest risk of gallstones (Maclure et al. 1989). The concentration of bile and subsequent stone formation during rapid weight loss, such as with an extremely low-calorie protein-sparing fast, are well documented. Drinking two to three cups of coffee daily reduced the risk of gallstones in men over a ten-year period (Leitzmann et al. 1999). High-glycemic foods that raise insulin levels also increase the risk of gallstones, so keeping to the low-glycemic type diet is helpful in preventing gallstones. Several supplements also can be useful to reduce bile cholesterol concentration.

STANDARD THERAPY

Gallstones are best diagnosed by ultrasound imaging of the upper abdomen. The most typical symptom of gallbladder disease is biliary colic, a condition of episodic sharp, cramping pain in the right upper quadrant. Liver damage can be suspected from abnormal liver function tests and encourages surgical remedy. Stones can be dislodged from the gallbladder and pass into the common bile duct, causing obstruction and jaundice (yellowing of skin and eyes from bile buildup in the blood), which almost always requires surgical intervention.

Laparoscopic surgery has been perfected in the past couple of decades and is minimally invasive with a brief recovery time compared to previous open gallbladder procedures. This is the procedure of choice. Bile salt therapy can be used to dissolve small stones, though therapy is prolonged and recurrence is common. Extracorporeal shock-wave therapy (*lithotripsy*) is a method in which larger stones can be broken into smaller fragments; stone recurrence also may be a problem. Some other rarely used techniques include dissolving stones with a potent cholesterol solvent, methyl tert-butyl ether (MTBE), and the use of monoterpenes (Rowachol) alone or in combination with bile salt therapy.

INTEGRATIVE APPROACHES

Integrative approaches are best reserved for patients with small or mildly symptomatic stones. Also they can be considered for those for whom surgery is not desired or is contraindicated. Botanical herbs can be used to stimulate bile flow (milk thistle, dandelion, artichoke) or to help dissolve small stones (peppermint oil). Diets deficient in vitamin C also promote gallstone formation. Calcium can help bind bile acids in the gut to reduce risk of gallstone formation. Lecithin can reduce levels of cholesterol in bile, so it can also be preventive (Tuzhilin et al. 1976).

Condition	Lifestyle Options	Conventional Medical/ Surgical Approaches	Botanical and Nutritional Supplements	Other Integrative, Functional, Holistic Solutions
Gallstones	For prevention: • Gradual weight loss and regular exercise • Low saturated-fat diet • Vegetarian diet • High-fiber diet • Drinking eight glasses of water daily • Reducing simple sugars in diet If you already have gallstones: • avoid raw vegetables. • Beets, dandelion greens, artichokes, and olive oil all improve bile flow.	• Diagnostic imaging with ultrasound • Liver function testing to detect damage done from gallstones obstructing outflow of liver • Laparoscopic cholecystectomy (removal of gallbladder using a scope and surgical instruments through small incisions in the abdomen) • Ursodiol-ursodeoxycholic acid / Actigall to help dissolve small (less than 1 cm) stones • Shock-wave therapy (*lithotripsy*) to break down stones	• Artichoke (1 to 4 g of leaf, stem, or root three times daily) • Dandelion (2 to 8 g dried root or 4 to 10 g of dried leaf three times daily, or make tea from these) • Lecithin (1000 mg twice daily) • Milk thistle (150 mg two to three times daily) • Peppermint oil (one to two enteric-coated capsules, 0.2 ml per cap three times a day) for dissolving small stones • Vitamin C (250 mg twice daily)	• Drink two to three cups of coffee daily. • If you have had your gallbladder removed, take bile salts to help deal with digestive issues and diarrhea.

Biochemical Factories Gone Amok: Liver and Pancreas

Hepatitis is an inflammation of the liver, usually caused by an infection, most commonly hepatitis virus A, B, or C; toxins such as alcohol, acetaminophen, or other drugs; or autoimmune causes.

Pancreatic insufficiency is a result of chronic pancreatitis from injury to the pancreas due to alcohol, trauma, viral infection, autoimmunity, obstruction, or other systemic causes.

RISK AND SIGNIFICANCE

The acute phase of hepatitis may resolve with no long-term consequences (this is common with hepatitis A or toxin-induced hepatitis, as from alcohol or drugs, when the inciting factor is removed). However, chronic liver disease is not uncommon and can be quite serious. Carrier states of the hepatitis B and C virus can cause chronic inflammation and damage to the liver, leading to cirrhosis and liver cancer. Chronic ingestion of alcohol in large quantities can likewise lead to progressive scarring, cirrhosis, and end-stage liver disease.

Chronic pancreatitis leads to pancreatic insufficiency. This causes malabsorption and the inability to digest food, particularly fats and fat-soluble vitamins. The exocrine pancreas, which secretes the digestive enzymes that break down protein, fat, and carbohydrates, is most often affected. However, the endocrine pancreas, which secretes insulin, can also be damaged, resulting in diabetes.

PREVENTION AND LIFESTYLE

Chronic liver disease is best avoided rather than treated. Healthy lifestyle options include reduction of exposure to toxins and infectious agents. Care needs to be taken particularly with alcohol and avoidance of IV drug use. Diets rich in antioxidants, even those found in tea and coffee, can support liver health (Ruhl and Everhart 2005). Chronic pancreatitis can also be prevented through similar healthy measures. Avoiding smoking is helpful in both conditions.

Vaccination plays an important role in preventing complications due to chronic liver disease. Health care workers and others who are more likely to be exposed are generally given the hepatitis B vaccine to prevent accidental infections.

STANDARD THERAPY

A number of advances have been made in the treatment of chronic infectious hepatitis B and C. These primarily include chemotherapy in the form of an immune booster, interferon, and an antiviral. Risk stratification for both conditions and likelihood of responding to therapy is complex and beyond the scope of this book. If you have hepatitis B or C, consultation with an expert in liver disease is essential. Some people, for example, do not require medication, as their own immune system is able to contain the condition and maintain the virus in a low level. Age, viral load, immune status, degree of damage to the liver as noted on biopsy, and the genotype of the virus are all factors considered in the treatment equation. Treatment is prolonged, almost a year in most cases, and not every person responds adequately.

Chronic pancreatic insufficiency may require managing persistent abdominal pain if there is ongoing chronic pancreatitis. The major GI problem with this condition is malabsorption. This is characterized by diarrhea or fatty, foul-smelling, and hard-to-flush stools containing undigested food. Mainstays of treatment are controlling the diarrhea, binding bile in the gut to reduce diarrhea and improve fat absorption, and replacement of digestive enzymes and unabsorbed nutrients (Mossner 1993).

Close monitoring of blood levels of calcium is necessary, especially when vitamin D is being replaced, as the levels of calcium may become too high.

INTEGRATIVE APPROACHES

In many cases, these conditions (chronic hepatitis and pancreatic insufficiency) do not respond to standard therapy and become lifelong conditions. While regular medical care must always be coupled with management, there are limits to standard approaches. This is when complementary therapies are a reasonable consideration. For example, in the acute phase after pancreatitis, substantial deficiencies of various vitamins and minerals occur, requiring repletion levels of these that then may subsequently be reduced. When and how to do this requires close medical monitoring, and the doses are adjusted according to individual needs and condition stage (Scolapio, Malhi-Chowla, and Ukleja 1999).

Long-term care then focuses on supporting the function of the chemical factory of the liver or pancreas to optimize digestive functions and to protect the organ from further harm. Antioxidants have been found to reduce free-radical damage in both conditions and are recommended by integrative practitioners (Kirk et al. 2006; Loguercio and Federico 2003; Andreone, Gramonzi, and Bernardi 1998). Of course, food sources ought to provide many of these antioxidants, but if food is not being absorbed or digested well, supplements are necessary. A number of herbs have been used traditionally for support of liver health. The most popular of these is milk thistle, which may help to protect against further damage to liver cells and help in regeneration. Additional immune support may be provided by schisandra, astragalus, and mushroom extracts, all of which have a long tradition of use in traditional Chinese medicine for liver and immune support. Consultation with an expert in Chinese medicine is an option for more complicated herbal formulas.

Scientific study supporting the use of most herbal medicines is not as robust as evidence-based medicine would demand. An experienced professional may be the best guide for using herbs and supplements to support liver health. Most physicians treating hepatitis with chemotherapy recommend avoiding herbal therapy during the interferon and antiviral therapy period, though the reasons for this are far from clear.

In pancreatic insufficiency, both conventional and integrative approaches attempt to manage nutrient deficiency, and such replacement needs to be monitored closely. The acute phase of replacement is generally one to four weeks, followed by maintenance therapy. Enzyme replacement is essential in pancreatic insufficiency to help with the absorption of nutrients and digestion of food, especially fat. A low-fat diet is recommended in most cases, except perhaps when the gut has been altered or shortened during surgery. Diabetes can be a consequence of pancreatic insufficiency and is treated with a combination of diet, exercise, and medications.

Condition	Lifestyle Options	Conventional Medical/ Surgical Approaches	Botanical and Nutritional Supplements	Other Integrative, Functional, Holistic Solutions
Chronic hepatitis	• Avoiding alcohol, acetaminophen, and other drugs and botanicals known to affect the liver • Reducing other toxins in diet or environment, such as tobacco, fumes, solvents, formaldehyde, pesticides, herbicides, and other xenobiotics • Avoiding intravenous drugs • Increasing antioxidant and detoxification potential (improving glutathione) status with asparagus, avocados, broccoli, spinach, garlic • Increasing fruit consumption • Regular exercise • Maintaining healthy body weight	Hepatitis B or C: • Abstinence from alcohol • Vaccination with hepatitis A and B if not immune • Vaccination with influenza annually, pneumococcal every five years, tetanus-diphtheria every ten years • Liver biopsy may be indicated • Screening for esophageal varices in cirrhosis patients • Screening for liver cancer • Liver transplant Hepatitis B: interferon (standard and pegylated), plus an antiviral such as lamivudine, adefovir dipivoxil, telbivudine, entecavir, or tenofovir Hepatitis C: pegylated interferon plus ribavirin for HCV genotype likely to have higher response (for example with genotypes 2 and 3 compared with 1)	• Antioxidants: vitamin C (250 mg twice daily and up to 3000 mg total); vitamin E (800 IU daily of mixed tocopherols); N-acetylcysteine (800 mg a day); lipoic acid (300 mg twice daily) • Astragalus (4 to 7 g of powder daily) • Milk thistle (210 mg two to three times a day as silymarin component) • Licorice root (250 to 500 mg dry powder three times daily or 1 to 2 g powdered root three times daily) • Mushrooms: maitake (7 g a day), shiitake (6 to 16 g a day), or reishi (1 to 9 g a day) whole dried mushrooms or in soup or tea. May also use liquid extracts (1 to 3 ml daily). Can use single or combined mushrooms. • Schisandra (100 mg of extract twice daily) • S-adenosylmethionine (SAM-e) (1600 mg a day) • Selenium (200 mg a day for immune boosting)	• Reduction of stress in lifestyle • Relaxation/ meditative techniques • Green tea (two to three cups daily) • Consider consultation with Chinese medical practitioner or other herbalist experienced with hepatitis B or C for individualized herbal mixtures.

Condition	Lifestyle Options	Conventional Medical/ Surgical Approaches	Botanical and Nutritional Supplements	Other Integrative, Functional, Holistic Solutions
Pancreatic insufficiency	• Abstaining from alcohol • Quitting smoking • Low-fat diet • Limiting caffeine to once daily to avoid worsening diarrhea • Consider diluting fruit juices or sugary drinks 1:1 with water	• Low-fat diet • Diarrhea: diphenoxylate with atropine/ Lomotil (one to two tabs after loose stool, not to exceed eight per day); loperamide/Imodium (2 to 4 mg as needed, not to exceed 16 mg a day) • Bile binding: cholestyramine (4 g three times daily); colestipol granules (5 to 10 g three times daily) • Pancreatic enzymes: Pancrelipase delayed-release capsules with meals; pancrelipase tablets and powder (1 g equivalent to 20000 units lipase component with meals)	• Vitamin C (250 mg twice daily and up to 3000 mg total); vitamin E (800 IU daily of mixed tocopherols or vitamin E as alpha-tocopheryl polyethylene glycol succinate) for severe fat malabsorption • Calcium carbonate (500 mg twice daily) • Ferrous gluconate (325 mg three times daily initially, then once daily) • Folic acid (5 mg daily in acute phase, then 1 mg daily) • Magnesium gluconate (350 to 500 mg four times daily acutely, then twice daily unless it aggravates diarrhea, then reduce) • Vitamin A (40000 to 50000 units twice daily acutely, then 8000 to 1000 units daily) • Vitamin B12 (1 mg subcutaneously up to three times weekly, then monthly; may also take sublingually or orally at 50 to 100 mcg daily for maintenance) • Vitamin D3 (30000 to 50000 units daily in acute recovery, then 2000 IU daily) • Vitamin K (2.5 to 12.5 mg daily)	• Control diabetes if present

The Unhappy Gut: Irritable Bowel Syndrome

Irritable bowel syndrome (IBS) is a condition characterized by chronic abdominal pain, bloating, distension, diarrhea, and/or constipation with no identifiable organic disorder.

RISK AND SIGNIFICANCE

IBS remains in many ways a medical mystery. It is predominantly a disease of women, found in 15 to 25 percent of women in Western society. The cause is unknown, and it remains a diagnosis of exclusion of other medical conditions. IBS has been associated with a number of conditions, such as food allergy or food intolerance, stress and anxiety, and a history of physical or sexual abuse. Motility of the gut may be increased, leading to the diarrhea variant, or slow, leading to constipation. Evacuation often relieves symptoms, at least temporarily. It is a troubling, uncomfortable condition but is benign, as it does not progress to more serious disease.

PREVENTION AND LIFESTYLE

General measures to reduce the impact of IBS on your life and health include attention to food intolerances or allergies, regular physical activity, stress management, and identification and treatment of post-traumatic stress disorder. Fiber intake is generally prescribed for IBS sufferers, but in some cases this may make the condition worse, possibly because of fermentation of undigested fiber in the gut (King 1998), leading to more gas and distension. You can try low amounts of different kinds of either soluble or insoluble fiber to see which works for your gut. Flaxseed bran or ground flaxseed is a favorite, particularly with constipation-variant IBS. Lactose, fructose, and sorbitol have been found to trigger IBS symptoms as well (Bohmer and Tuynman 1996). So if you notice increased symptoms after consuming any of these in your diet, eliminate them.

STANDARD THERAPY

In many ways, standard and integrative therapies converge in the management of IBS. A remarkable study found that the therapeutic relationship had a significant positive placebo effect in IBS (Kaptchuk et al. 2008). Subjects who experienced warmth, attention, and confidence from their care provider did significantly better than a "placebo" (standard care) group, who did better than a group on a waiting list.

Beyond this, it is essential that you identify dietary and lifestyle factors that aggravate the condition. Roughly, recommendations for care can be stratified into mild, moderate, and severe symptoms. In mild cases, reassurance, dietary modification, and fiber are all that is usually necessary. If you are moderately symptomatic, there is more focus on food intolerances, psychological counseling, and stress management. Medications for both acute relief and long-term symptom management are utilized. For severe, intractable cases, strong consideration is given to the psychological issues likely to be underlying IBS, such as a history of sexual abuse. Counseling and mood-altering medications, as well as pharmaceuticals for symptom relief, are added.

INTEGRATIVE APPROACHES

If you suffer from IBS, compassion, patience, and understanding from both care providers and significant others undergird the integrative approach (Spanier, Howden, and Jones 2003). It is essential that you understand the chronic-though-benign nature of the condition, empower your ability to participate in making healthy lifestyle and treatment decisions, and consider the full range of potential triggering or aggravating factors. Making a food diary to track symptoms is usually productive. You may want to try a variety of relaxation and stress management techniques and, if needed, professional counseling (Lackner et al. 2007; Dancey, Taghavi, and Fox 1998; Waxman 1988).

Additional measures are a variety of herbals that can relax the gut and reduce spasm and pain, along with increasing fiber and eliminating offending foods (Liu et al. 2006; Pittler and Ernst 1998). Probiotics have been found useful in many who suffer with IBS (Kajander et al. 2008; Whorwell et al. 2007; Spiller 2005). Acupuncture is also highly effective in some people and is both safe and simple. Traditional Chinese herbs have also been proven to be useful, particularly when individualized to a specific patient (Bensoussan et al. 1998).

Condition	Lifestyle Options	Conventional Medical/Surgical Approaches	Botanical and Nutritional Supplements	Other Integrative, Functional, Holistic Solutions
Irritable bowel syndrome	• High-fiber foods • Treating food allergy if present • Identifying lactose and/or fructose intolerance • Getting regular light to moderate exercise • Paleolithic (caveman) diet with less grains or processed foods	• Develop a positive therapeutic relationship • Patient education • Psychological therapies (see other integrative, functional, holistic solutions) • Dietary modification: lactose, gluten, carbohydrates, food allergy, gas-producing foods • Fiber (insoluble vs. soluble): psyllium, wheat bran or polycarbophil, methylcellulose (trial of one-half to one tablespoon daily to start) • Antispasmodics (as needed): dicyclomine/Bentyl (20 mg up to four times daily); hyoscyamine/Levsin (0.125 to 0.25 mg three or four times daily); sustained release hyoscyamine/Levbid (0.375 to 0.75 mg every twelve hours) • Antidepressants (any of these may be considered particularly with coexisting depression): amitriptyline, desipramine, imipramine, nortriptyline (dosing is variable based on response and side effects, such as constipation); paroxetine (20 mg daily); fluoxetine (20 mg daily); sertraline (100 mg PO daily) • Anti-diarrheals: loperamide/Imodium (2 to 4 mg as needed, not to exceed 16 mg a day) • Anxiolytics for short-term use only for acute anxiety: lorazepam/Ativan (0.5 to 1 mg up to three times daily); diazepam/Valium (1 to 10 mg up to three times daily); oxazepam/Serza (10 to 30 mg three times daily) • Serotonin antagonists for relief of abdominal pain and discomfort: ondansetron/Zofran (4 to 8 mg one to two times daily; granisetron/Granisol (2 mg daily) • Other: lubiprostone/Amitiza (8 mcg twice daily for women over eighteen with constipation-variety IBS)	• Peppermint oil (one to two enteric-coated capsules three times daily) • Caraway oil: enteric-coated volatile oil (0.05 to 0.2 ml can be taken three times daily); can be taken in combination with peppermint oil • Fennel (one teaspoon with food), also available as tea, oil capsule, alcohol extract • Ginger (250 to 500 mg three to four times daily, or as tea, one cup before meals) • Chamomile (one cup of tea three times daily)	• Relaxation exercises • Management of stress and anxiety • Cognitive behavioral therapy • Hypnotherapy • Biofeedback • Psychotherapy • Mindful eating • Probiotics (up to 25 billion units of *Bifidobacteria* and 25 billion units of *Lactobacillus* for four to six weeks then 10 BU daily, mixed species) • Soluble fiber, such as psyllium, ground flaxseed two to three tablespoons daily • Iberogast (twenty drops three times a day for four weeks) • Rifamixin (400 mg three times daily) for small intestinal bacterial overgrowth • Avoid or limit antibiotics to prevent dysbiosis. • Consider acupuncture.

Gut on Fire: Inflammatory Bowel Disease

Inflammatory bowel disease (IBD) refers to chronic, relapsing, inflammatory conditions of the bowel with unknown cause. Crohn's disease (CD) can involve any part of the bowel, including the stomach, small bowel, and colon. Ulcerative colitis (UC) affects primarily the colon and rectum.

RISK AND SIGNIFICANCE

Both CD and UC are major and serious GI conditions characterized by diarrhea, bleeding and mucus in the stools, abdominal pain, and many potential complications. These complications include infection, bowel obstruction, colon cancer, and symptoms outside the gut such as arthritis. Both seem to have genetic tendencies, as they run in families and are seen more commonly in Jewish people. Breast-feeding as an infant seems to be protective against inflammatory bowel disease. Cigarette smoking actually seems to protect against UC but increases the risk of CD. Anti-inflammatory drugs (NSAIDs and COX-2s) have been implicated in at least some cases of inflammatory bowel disease, as have oral contraceptives. Association with food and food allergy is less clear. Living in a southern climate or a less developed country seems to decrease risk, suggesting that environment plays a role in the occurrence of these conditions.

PREVENTION AND LIFESTYLE

Data are controversial here, though some experts recommend an anti-inflammatory diet, addressing possible food allergy (Candy et al. 1995), and minimizing alcohol. Breast-feeding your children lowers their risk of inflammatory bowel disease. Regular colonoscopy is strongly advised in UC since UC is associated with a major increase in the risk of colon cancer.

STANDARD THERAPY

Standard medical approaches are the mainstay of these conditions and include multiple types of potent anti-inflammatory drugs, steroids, immunosuppressants, and sometimes surgery. Management is best directed by a physician who has expertise in medical treatments and who knows how best to balance the potency and risk of the treatment with the severity of the disease.

INTEGRATIVE APPROACHES

Given the seriousness of both of these conditions, you should consider all possible options, as well as consult with your trusted medical professional. General principles include reducing inflammation with an anti-inflammatory diet and supplements such as aloe, boswellia, curcumin, omega-3 fatty acids, glutamine, and wheat grass (Langmead et al. 2004; Gupta et al. 1997; Hanai et al. 2006; Aslan and Triadafilopoulos 1992; Ben-Arye et al. 2002). Many studies have examined the benefits of fish oil (Dichi et al. 2000; Belluzzi et al. 1996; Stenson et al. 1992), and I recommend it as well. Malabsorption of essential vitamins and minerals requires replacement to support healing and the immune response. Bone loss prevention requires vitamin D and calcium (Vogelsang et al. 1995). Antioxidants can also reduce free-radical damage from inflammation.

Probiotics have a mixed track record, and though they have been used in high doses with success, particularly in UC in children and infection of surgical pouches in UC, they need to be used carefully. Start with low doses and gradually increase to a clinical effect, such as decreased diarrhea, pain, or bleeding. Many recent studies support the beneficial role of probiotics in IBD (Fujimori et al. 2009; Vanderpool, Yan, and Polk 2008; Mallon et al. 2007; Rolfe et al. 2006; Bohm and Kruis 2006; Tamboli et al. 2004). Implantation of normal gut flora by enema in patients with UC has even been found to be helpful (Borody et al. 2003; Bennet and Brinkman 1989). Stay tuned.

Stress management is helpful, as these conditions impose significant burdens on your day-to-day life. A couple of good books to help you explore alternatives to conventional therapy are *Breaking the Vicious Cycle* and *The New Eating Right for a Bad Gut* (see resources). If you decide to use complementary treatments outside the standard therapy approach, be sure to choose a skilled holistic practitioner and a dietician as your guides.

Condition	Lifestyle Options	Conventional Medical/Surgical Approaches	Botanical and Nutritional Supplements	Other Integrative, Functional, Holistic Solutions
Inflammatory bowel disease: Crohn's disease and ulcerative colitis	• Maintaining an anti-inflammatory diet • Identifying food allergy • Minimizing alcohol intake	Crohn's disease: • Mesalamine/Pentasa or Asacol (2 g a day with an increase to a maximum of 4.8 g a day) • Sulfasalazine/Asacol (2 to 4 g daily) • Prednisone (40 to 60 mg daily for ten to fourteen days, then decrease) • Budesonide/Entocort EC (8 mg daily for eight weeks then decrease to 6 mg for up to three months) • Immunosuppressant therapy, such as infliximab, adalimumab, certolizumab pegol • Azathioprine or 6-mercaptopurine • Antibiotics, such as metronidazole, quinolones • Surgery: multiple types including removal of sections of bowel, ileostomy, treatment of infection, strictures, fistulas Ulcerative colitis: • Sulfasalazine/Azulfidine, mesalamine/Pentasa, Asacol, Lialda, Apriso, olsalazine/Dipentum, or balsalazide/Colazal: local application as enemas and suppositories for rectal or left-sided colon problems; systemic dosing for nonresponsive or more extensive disease to maximum tolerated and then lowered to maintenance (dosages vary per drug) • Steroids: prednisone and budesonide as above in CD • Immunosuppressive therapy: cyclosporine, infliximab, methotrexate, azathioprine, mercaptopurine • Surgery: colectomy (removal of part or all of colon), multiple variations with and without colostomy	• Aloe (half cup three times daily) • Rice bran oil (100 mg three times daily for three to six weeks) • Boswellia (550 mg three times daily) • Curcumin (1 g twice daily) • Fish oil (6 g daily at least 3.2 g EPA and 2.2 g DHA) • Glutamine (1600 to 3000 mg daily in three to four divided doses) • Wheat grass juice (three and a half ounces daily for a month) • Supplements to replace malabsorbed nutrients, i.e., calcium (1200 mg/day), magnesium (350 mg/day), iron (300 mg/day), selenium (200 mcg/day), zinc (30 mg/day), vitamins A (5000 IU/day), B1 (50 mg/day), B6 (50 mg/day), folic acid (400 mcg/day), B12 (50 mcg/day), Vitamin D (2000 IU daily) • Antioxidants such as beta carotenoids (10000 IU daily), vitamin C (250 to 500 mg daily), CoQ10 (50 to 100 mg daily)	• Stress management • Probiotics: mixed species (start with low dose of 1 BU three times daily and gradually increase over a month to 20 to 30 BU daily; some UC patients have safely taken as much as 200 to 500 BU daily) • Saccharomyces boulardii (250 mg three times daily) for CD diarrhea • Nicotine patches (UC)

Pockets of Pain: Diverticulosis

Diverticulosis is a condition in which there are small outpocketings or sac-like protrusions of the bowel, usually the colon. These may not cause symptoms unless they get blocked, infected, or inflamed. In this case, they create diverticulitis, a condition that can cause pain, fever, infection, abscess formation, and bleeding.

RISK AND SIGNIFICANCE

Diverticular disease seems to be a condition of Western civilization. While countries in Africa and Asia have an incidence of under 0.2 percent, the United States and other developed nations have rates up to 45 percent. Asians adopting a more Western lifestyle and diet have a similar rate as that seen with the U.S. population. This suggests important environmental and lifestyle issues contribute to this condition (Etzioni et al. 2009). Diverticulosis and diverticulitis have traditionally been seen primarily in older persons, with rates of up to 65 percent in those eighty-five or older. However, more recently, rates of this condition as measured by hospital admissions for diverticulitis have jumped substantially in the eighteen to forty-four age group. This could be you. The risk of colon cancer is increased in those with diverticulosis (Etzioni et al. 2009; Acosta et al. 1992).

PREVENTION AND LIFESTYLE

A high-fiber diet is an established protective factor for diverticulosis. You should ingest at least 25 grams of fiber daily. Interestingly, vegetarians seem to have less diverticulosis, probably because fruits and vegetables have much higher amounts of fiber (Aldoori et al. 1994). Passing large-bore stools improves segmental colon activity and is a likely factor in reducing the risk of diverticular disease. Remember the motto to try to pass "fluffy floaters" not "sinking slinkers." More fiber is good. This fiber issue likely accounts for the difference in the occurrence of diverticulosis in developed versus underdeveloped countries. We are being out-pooped in terms of the bulk and caliber of our stool due to our lower fiber intake.

Obesity and lack of physical activity have also been found to contribute to the prevalence of diverticulosis (Aldoori et al. 1995). Constipation is also a likely contributor to diverticulosis, though in clinical studies this has been hard to prove, no pun intended. Simple physics describing wall tension and muscular contraction, however, predict diverticula occurring at areas of colon-wall weakness, where blood vessels penetrate, so constipation is a logical risk factor.

STANDARD THERAPY

Treatment for diverticulosis is primarily the maintenance of a high-fiber diet. This reduces pressure in the bowel and reduces the risk of acute diverticulitis. Conventional wisdom has long recommended avoiding small food items, such as seeds, nuts, and popcorn. It was thought that they would lodge in the diverticula, causing blockage and inflammation, but this has now been disputed. In fact, an eighteen-year study of men with diverticular disease who ate popcorn, corn, and nuts actually showed a lower incidence of diverticulitis (Strate et al. 2008).

In acute attacks of diverticulitis, the person is usually afflicted with abdominal pain, most commonly in the left lower abdomen, though it can occur elsewhere along the course of the colon. It is important to exclude other problems, such as appendicitis, gallbladder disease, or colon cancer, and then for the doctor to determine if the attack is uncomplicated or complicated. In routine, uncomplicated cases with just abdominal tenderness and some fever, therapy as an outpatient with clear fluids for three days and oral antibiotics is adequate. If you do not respond and have increased fever, have abdominal pain, or are unable to take fluids, you may need to be admitted to the hospital. With complicated diverticulitis, you may have evidence of abscess, fistula, bleeding, perforation, or obstruction on physical examination or X-ray. CT scans of the abdomen are very useful in detecting such complications, which may require not only admission to the hospital for IV antibiotics but also surgery.

Follow-up studies in two to six weeks following an acute attack are recommended, to exclude more serious conditions like cancer. In up to 30 percent of instances, even uncomplicated cases can benefit from surgery after the first attack (Stollman and Raskin 1999).

INTEGRATIVE APPROACHES

Most integrative approaches in diverticular disease are aimed at preventing it in the first place or reducing the risk of acute inflammation. Options for managing uncomplicated cases include supplements like rice bran oil, glutamine, and slippery elm bark to help heal the colon. If there is significant pain and fever, I recommend antibiotics. Probiotics may also have a role in decreasing intestinal inflammation and infection. I prefer flaxseed bran as a form of fiber because of its high omega-3 content and anti-inflammatory properties.

Condition	Lifestyle Options	Conventional Medical/Surgical Approaches	Botanical and Nutritional Supplements	Other Integrative, Functional, Holistic Solutions
Diverticulosis	• Preventing with high-fiber, low-fat diet • Avoiding constipation using fiber, stool softeners • Getting regular physical activity such as running • It is no longer universally recommended to avoid small seeds and nuts	Uncomplicated (abdominal pain, fever): • Outpatient therapy • Clear liquids for three days • Antibiotics: ciprofloxacin/Cipro (500 mg twice daily); metronidazole/Flagyl (500 mg three times daily). Other options for those intolerant of these medications are amoxicillin-clavulanate, clindamycin, or moxifloxacin • Restart high-fiber diet when acute condition subsides. • Colonoscopy two to six weeks after acute episode to exclude cancer or other disease • Up to 30 percent of uncomplicated cases require surgery. Complicated (high fever, severe abdominal pain, bleeding, obstruction, perforation, abscess, fistula formation): • Admit to hospital for IV fluids and antibiotics (multiple possible combinations) • CT scan • Consider surgery emergently or after initial treatment • Colonoscopy two to six weeks after acute episode to exclude cancer or other disease	• Rice bran oil (100 mg three times daily for three to six weeks) • Glutamine (up to 8 g daily in three to four divided doses, adjusted according to response) • Slippery elm bark (one to two capsules three times daily, or make a tea with one teaspoon in two cups of water and use freely)	• Soluble fiber such as psyllium, ground flaxseed (two to three tablespoons daily) • Probiotics to prevent infection: *acidophilus/Bifidobacteria* (one capsule twice daily for prevention, two capsules three times daily during flare-ups)

Pain in the... Hemorrhoids

Hemorrhoids are normal veins within the anal canal, of concern only when they cause symptoms. These symptoms can be bleeding, itching, pain, prolapse (pouching out of rectum), or thrombosis (a hemorrhoid containing a swollen blood clot).

RISK AND SIGNIFICANCE

Traditionally, hemorrhoids have been associated with pregnancy, prolonged sitting or standing, increased age, family history, diarrhea, straining, and pelvic area tumors. Recent studies have disputed the long-standing belief that hemorrhoids are associated with chronic constipation, though this remains controversial (Johanson and Sonnenberg 1990, 1994). The main problems with hemorrhoids are symptoms of discomfort, bleeding, and itching. While hemorrhoids are a very common source of rectal bleeding, even in younger people, those over forty should be evaluated further for such problems as diverticulosis, *angiodysplasia* (abnormal blood vessels in the intestine and colon), inflammatory bowel disease or infection, and malignancy.

PREVENTION AND LIFESTYLE

Though the association of hemorrhoids and constipation has been questioned, it is still prudent to maintain a high-fiber diet and avoid straining at stool. Prolonged sitting or standing can be a contributing factor, so occupations that require this, such as truck driver, waitress, or surgeon, may make you more prone to both hemorrhoids and their near cousin, varicose veins of the legs. Both conditions are due to increased venous congestion. Physical activity is considered helpful, though some kinds of exercise, such as weight lifting, may aggravate hemorrhoids because of increased abdominal pressure. Obesity may also contribute to hemorrhoids, so weight loss is recommended if you are overweight. A high-fiber diet and good fluid intake are also preventive.

STANDARD THERAPY

Fluid, fiber, and topical treatments are the initial approaches to symptomatic hemorrhoids. Witch hazel–impregnated pads such as Tucks can be soothing and will help with cleansing of the anus and rectal area. Protruding or bulky hemorrhoids can make adequate hygiene of this area difficult, so such pads are useful. Once you have cleansed the irritated hemorrhoidal tissue and anus, putting 1 percent hydrocortisone cream on one of the witch hazel pads and applying it liberally to the area has an anti-inflammatory effect. For internal hemorrhoids, suppositories containing Peruvian balsam and hydrocortisone can be very soothing. Sitz baths (baths with salts such as Epsom salts) are also helpful for cleansing and pain relief, as is the use of a bidet. Stool softeners can be useful both to lessen the pain of defecation and to prevent further irritation.

Sometimes, surgical measures are needed. The thrombosed hemorrhoid (a blood clot in an internal or external hemorrhoid) is to be suspected if you feel a sudden lump, the size and consistency of a grape, accompanied by pain in the rectal area. If you can see a doctor within forty-eight hours of its appearance, a simple office procedure to open the clotted hemorrhoid provides immediate relief. Beyond that time, the clot starts to resolve and organize into scar tissue, and measures like baths, pain medications, and local creams can help. Surgical removal may be useful later.

More advanced or recurrent hemorrhoids can be treated with a large number of minimally invasive or advanced surgical techniques. Your physician or surgeon can guide you to the best approach.

INTEGRATIVE APPROACHES

In addition to lifestyle measures, such as baths, fiber (Alonso-Coello et al. 2006), and stool softeners, a number of botanical and nutritional products can be useful. Horse chestnut, butcher's broom, and flavonoids can be taken by mouth to reduce pain and inflammation in hemorrhoidal tissue (Misra and Parshad 2000). These products are also available topically to apply to inflamed tissue instead of using hydrocortisone. Topical witch hazel is very helpful, as described above.

Condition	Lifestyle Options	Conventional Medical/ Surgical Approaches	Botanical and Nutritional Supplements	Other Integrative, Functional, Holistic Solutions
Hemorrhoids	• Increasing fiber in diet • Treating constipation with stool softeners • Maintaining active exercise program • Maintaining high fluid intake (at least sixty-four ounces water daily) • Losing weight • Taking warm sitz baths two to three times daily during flares (may alternate warm and cold baths); add Epsom salts for cleansing, astringent effects	• Conservative treatment with fiber, increased fluids • Application of topical hydrocortisone for up to a week with pain and itching • Lancing and draining of thrombosed (clotted) hemorrhoids if less than forty-eight hours old • Minimally invasive surgical treatments: banding, coagulation, injection with sclerosing agent, cryotherapy • Hemorrhoidectomy with surgical scalpel, diathermy, laser, ultrasonic scalpel, or stapling for more extensive or severely prolapsed hemorrhoids • Colonoscopy for those over forty with rectal bleeding to exclude other causes of GI bleeding besides hemorrhoids, such as colon cancer, diverticulitis	• Horse chestnut (300 mg two to three times a day) • Bioflavonoid complex (1000 mg three times a day during flares) • Butcher's broom (100 mg three times daily) • Application of topical gels or creams containing 2 percent aescin (active ingredient in horse chestnut) • Topical witch hazel	• Soluble fiber such as psyllium, ground flaxseed (one to three tablespoons daily)

CONCLUSION

So now you have become an expert in matters pertaining to maintaining a healthy gut. As you can see, there are many things you can do for yourself in terms of prevention and lifestyle as well as treatment. Consider the prescriptions and recommendations in this chapter in the context of the whole book. Preventing and treating gut issues is a wide-ranging topic, including primary dietary and lifestyle measures and highly targeted drug therapies. In between are many herbs, supplements, and over-the-counter remedies that can spare you the pain of the scalpel or the cost and potential side effects of medications. Read on for further details.

Chapter 10

Don't Take Once
a Day Forever

Problems with Commonly
Used Medications

If you have a chronic GI problem, such as GERD, IBD, or IBS, you may require ongoing management with medication. It's important to tend to the rest of the body and be aware of the benefits and the unseen dangers of certain GI drugs. This chapter identifies the benefits and some of the risks associated with the most commonly used medications. It offers some lifestyle options that will help you keep drug use to a minimum, as well as some suggestions for how to best manage these drugs if you have to take them. For further discussion of holistic, functional, and integrative solutions to GI problems, see chapter 9.

COMMON GI DRUGS

The following table lists medications commonly used for gastrointestinal conditions, along with their benefits and their potential side effects and risks.

Condition	Medication	Effects	Potential Side Effects	Lifestyle Options
Gingivitis	Antibiotics	Treats infection	Allergic reactions, drug resistance, change in gut bacteria (dysbiosis)	Brush and floss regularly; avoid simple sugars
Esophagitis and gastroesophageal reflux disease	Antacids: Maalox, Mylanta, Gaviscon H2 blockers: ranitidine/Zantac, famotidine/Pepcid, cimetidine/Tagamet Proton pump inhibitors: omperazole/Prilosec, pantoprazole/Protonix, esomeprazole/Nexium, rabeparazole/Aciphex	Reduces the acidity level of stomach contents which back up into the esophagus. Cuts down symptoms of burning, spasm, asthma, risk of scarring, strictures, and esophageal cancer	Skin, blood, pancreas, and kidney problems; headache; diarrhea; abdominal pain; nausea; decreased absorption of nutrients, such as vitamin B12, calcium, magnesium, and others (PPIs); increased risk of infections (PPIs)	Eat smaller meals; elevate head of bed by six inches to reduce reflux; avoid offending foods and beverages; stop smoking; lose weight
Gastritis and ulcers	Antacids; sucralfate/Carafate; antibiotics to treat *H. pylori* infection; foaming agents	Reduces acid production in stomach. Coats stomach. Allows mucus production to help heal ulcers and inflammation. Reduces bacterial inflammation from *H. pylori* (antibiotics)	Skin, blood, pancreas, and kidney problems; headache; diarrhea; abdominal pain; nausea; decreased absorption of nutrients (PPIs); increased risk of infections (PPIs)	Avoid offending foods, beverages, and drugs (aspirin, steroids, NSAIDs like ibuprofen, naproxen, and others); manage stress

Condition	Medication	Effects	Potential Side Effects	Lifestyle Options
Irritable bowel syndrome	Antispasmodics	Reduces cramping and pain	Confusion; psychosis; blurred vision; urinary retention; dry mouth; headache; insomnia; rapid heartbeat, nausea; constipation; impotence; fever	Do relaxation exercises; manage stress and anxiety; eat high-fiber foods; treat food allergy if present
Inflammatory bowel disease	Steroids and other anti-inflammatories	Quiets inflammation; reduces bleeding, ulcerations	Steroids: adrenal suppression; hypertension; ulcers; weight gain; immune suppression; confusion; nervousness; psychosis; acne and other skin problems; worsening of diabetic control; edema; headache; insomnia; muscle weakness Sulfasalazine: skin rashes (mild to severe); lung, liver, kidney, blood problems; pancreatitis; headache; nausea/vomiting; stomach upset; blood in urine; fever	Maintain an anti-inflammatory diet
Diverticulosis	Antibiotics	Treats infection	Allergic reactions; drug resistance; changes in gut bacteria (dysbiosis)	Prevent with high-fiber diet; avoid constipation using fiber
Hemorrhoids	Topical agents like Preparation H; topical steroids	Reduces swelling; soothes inflamed tissue	Local irritation; burning; infection; allergic reaction	Lose weight; treat constipation with stool softeners; increase fiber in diet

Information on side effects abstracted from the *Physicians' Desk Reference* (2009) and Epocrates (2010).

While not comprehensive, the preceding table gives a range of benefits and problems that can come from common medications given for GI conditions. Medication may be enormously helpful, but you must be vigilant about the potential for side effects from taking these or any medications. This is particularly true if you are a person with allergies to foods, drugs, or other substances or if you have noted difficulty metabolizing medications in the past: frequent side effects, intolerance of standard dosing, and so on.

CAVEAT EMPTOR (LET THE BUYER BEWARE)

The following discussion examines more closely the potential benefits and side effects of taking some of the medications mentioned in the preceding table and makes some suggestions for how to minimize your reliance on these drugs where possible.

Proton Pump Inhibitors

The drugs in this class, commonly called PPIs, are powerful suppressors of acid. As you may recall from high school or college chemistry, the hydrogen ion is basically a proton and the building block in hydrochloric acid production. Hydrochloric acid is the primary digestive chemical in the stomach. Due to its very high acidity (pH around 2), it initiates the breakdown of foods. Unfortunately, this acid can turn against the stomach itself, causing irritation, inflammation, and ulceration. This can happen when the thick mucus lining or cells of the stomach aren't functioning properly, are unable to repair themselves because of drugs, foods, or other irritating substances, or are infected with *H. pylori*. In such cases, shutting down acid production with PPIs can be useful to relieve symptoms and promote healing.

PPIs are one of the most useful classes of medication that has been discovered in the last thirty years. They have drastically reduced the need for surgery for ulcers and other upper GI problems and are an important part of medical practice.

However, long-term suppression of normal stomach function might be expected to produce some adverse outcomes. In fact, the Food and Drug Administration has only approved the use of PPIs for an eight-week period, though some people take them daily for indefinite periods of time. The problem is that even if these drugs are tolerated, they can be associated with other adverse health issues. Since the listed side effects are not seen in everyone, many people are able to take these medicines long term with a sense of safety, but doing so may be at a cost to your health. Speaking of cost, such drugs can cost up to or more than $100 per month, depending on the dosage and insurance coverage. Even over-the-counter formulations can be expensive for a minimal daily dose.

Some potential problems from this potent acid suppression are increased intestinal infections and overgrowth of bacteria in the small bowel. Because stomach acid is a first line of defense against bacteria that we swallow, the absence of such acid has been shown to increase the occurrence of infections of the stomach, small intestine, and colon, and even pneumonia in the lung (Termanini et al. 1998; Selway 1990; Laheij et al. 2004). PPI drugs also reduce the absorption of calcium, iron, and vitamin B_{12}, which can lead to osteoporosis, certain kinds of anemia, and nerve problems. The chronic suppression of acid has been found to be associated with colorectal cancer (Robertson et al. 2007), and concerns persist regarding long-term risk of stomach cancer, though this has never been reported. Food allergy may also be increased because of decreased breakdown of proteins in the stomach, which then are presented downstream in undigested form to the gut's immune system (Untersmayr et al. 2003). Don't avoid these medications if you need them, but be aware of their risks.

THE PPI TAPER-OFF APPROACH

Once your acute condition, ulcer, reflux, or other problem has improved, it's a good idea to taper off the PPI and substitute with a less potent antacid, such as one of the H2 blockers. To do this, you would use the PPI and the H2 blocker on alternate days, observing whether symptoms recur and, if they don't, gradually reduce the PPI and replace it with the H2 blocker. If the less potent drug controls your symptoms adequately, then you keep the PPIs in reserve for flare-ups of your condition. For flare-ups, you can take the PPI for a couple of weeks or so, and taper off again. The PPIs don't work as quickly as H2 blockers or even other antacids, like Maalox or Mylanta; they take a couple of days to shut down acid production completely. Therefore, you may require one of the other types of antacids for temporary relief while restarting a PPI. Stopping a PPI abruptly may result in a rebound-increase in acidity, so tapering off is safer. Consult with your doctor or other health care provider about the taper regimen.

Antibiotics

One of the most surprising medical discoveries in the past few decades is that bacteria can cause stomach ulcers. The discovery of the bacterium *H. pylori* and its importance in ulcer disease has expanded the use of antibiotics for GI indications. The discoverers garnered a Nobel Prize for this important scientific advance. About 80 percent of stomach ulcers are caused by *H. pylori*, though this seems to be decreasing (Chiorean et al. 2002). This infection can also contribute to reflux disease and gastritis. Effective treatment requires at least two antibiotics plus a PPI. There are several other protocols, some involving bismuth (Pepto-Bismol), H2 blockers, and two antibiotics. This combined-drug approach is highly effective, although about 20 percent of the time ulcers recur within six months (Vakil 2005).

Other usages for antibiotics in GI problems are for bacterial infections of the colon, like infectious diarrhea, diverticulitis, and sometimes gallbladder inflammation.

Antibiotics are a powerful and highly useful—sometimes lifesaving—group of medications, but this expanded antibiotic use can cause problems. Though antibiotics are usually given for a short time, their effects can be long term. Chapter 3 discussed the impact of antibiotics on causing dysbiosis or alterations in gut bacteria with subsequent effects on immunity, food allergy, and infectious disease. A well-known problem with antibiotic usage is the overgrowth of another type of bacteria, *Clostridium difficile*, which causes a troublesome diarrhea. Treatment requires even more antibiotics to eliminate *C. difficile*, resulting in a further disruption in gut microbiota.

To offset the damage done by giving potent antibiotics for gut infections or superinfections, I recommend taking 10 to 30 billion units of mixed probiotics while on medication and for two to four weeks thereafter. This minimizes the risk of *C. difficile* and other dysbiotic infections and their secondary results. You should take the probiotic spaced as far away from the antibiotic as possible during therapy.

In addition to medical use, the presence of antibiotics in our food supply contributes to antibiotic resistance. A common practice is to feed chickens, cows, and other animals antibiotics to prevent infections as they are kept in crowded pens. This results in bacterial resistance being passed onto meat-eating humans or through offal runoff into rivers and streams as an environmental pollutant. Antibiotic allergy is quite common and can be serious. As we are exposed to more antibiotics in our medicines, food, and even water supply, the rate of allergy to antibiotics increases, raising the risk that when needed for a life-threatening condition, the best antibiotic might not be tolerated. I have a number of patients in this situation. Finding a suitable antibiotic that is safe, affordable, and effective can be a major challenge even for a routine respiratory, skin, or urinary tract infection.

You should take antibiotics when necessary, but be aware of potential negative consequences and avoid them when you can. Make this decision in consultation with your health care provider. Health professionals are more and more aware of the risks of overprescribing antibiotics in both children and adults.

Steroids and Anti-Inflammatory Drugs

One of the most common classes of drugs used over-the-counter these days is the non-steroidal anti-inflammatory drugs (NSAIDs). When I was a medical student, these potent drugs were considered dangerous enough to be available only by prescription. Currently, some NSAIDs, such as ibuprofen and naproxen, are available over the counter. Often, these drugs are taken daily for chronic conditions like arthritis or acutely for other pain, such as sprains, strains, fever, and inflammation. While often useful, these medications can cause ulceration and bleeding in the stomach, intestines, and colon. In fact, data shows that over 16,000 deaths occur annually in the United States as a result of taking NSAIDs, mostly among the elderly (Wolfe, Lichtenstein, and Singh 1999). Numerous hospitalizations are also attributed to these medications, which also may cause leaky gut syndrome.

As with other medications, you should take NSAIDs when needed, but exert caution since long-term use increases the risk of side effects and complications. The fact that you can obtain NSAIDs without a prescription doesn't necessarily mean that they are always safe for everyone.

Steroids, like prednisone, triamcinolone, dexamethasone, and prednisolone, have an even higher side effect profile in the gut and elsewhere. This class of drugs is broadly used for immune disorders, severe forms of arthritis, many skin conditions, asthma, allergies, nervous system disorders, pain conditions, and much more. Steroids are available as pills, shots, IV injections, inhalers and nasal sprays, and topical applications, such as skin creams and ointments. The oral and injectable forms have the most potent effect on the gut, while the other forms have much less or minimal effects. Steroids can cause ulcers and bleeding, diminish immunity, affect gut bacteria, and have other systemic effects. Sulfasalazine, which is a useful NSAID commonly used for inflammatory bowel disease, can have side effects similar to those associated with steroid use.

These drugs can be lifesaving and are sometimes the gastroenterologist's best friend. When taken long term, you must attend to their risks as well as benefits.

Anti-Spasmodics

This group of drugs is prescribed to reduce painful cramps and spasms in the intestine and stomach and to promote passage of food and digestive contents. Some people take these all the time and tolerate them well. A couple of drugs in this class (cisapride, Zelnorm) were removed from the market because of safety reasons related to the heart and other organs, but others remain available. All have potential for serious side effects. These include Parkinson-like symptoms, tremors, muscle twitches, confusion, and drowsiness. Use of these drugs must be tempered with caution, trading off the relief they offer with the risk for drug interactions and side effects.

CONCLUSION

The information in this chapter should help you make wise choices for your gut health. If you are taking or considering taking any medication, it's important to know about the potential side effects and to opt for lifestyle changes that may help to minimize your need for drugs. You may want to review chapter 9, which covers some holistic, nondrug therapies for your GI health. Many natural products, herbs, supplements, and over-the-counter products can be useful health options for acute and chronic GI conditions at less cost and less risk.

CHAPTER 11

A COMPREHENSIVE ELIMINATION DIET AND OTHER DELIGHTS

HIGH-FIBER AND DETOXIFICATION PLANS

Previous chapters have covered some of the issues related to food allergies and sensitivities. This chapter presents the best way to identify food allergies and sensitivities and in the process improve your gut and overall health. It also offers some tips on how to increase fiber in your diet and some helpful methods for cleansing and detoxification of your gut.

THE COMPREHENSIVE ELIMINATION DIET

If you believe that you may have food allergies or sensitivities, the following instructions will give you the best tool for assessing your various reactions to foods. Undertaking a comprehensive elimination diet requires a strong commitment from you. In the first half of this diet, you eliminate common and potentially offending foods; then you gradually test your response to specific foods as you reintroduce them into your diet. This can take several weeks or more to complete and be a major event both diagnostically and therapeutically. The following case study shows how the functional medicine approach and a comprehensive elimination diet worked for a former patient.

Trudy's Story

Trudy was a fifty-six-year-old who suffered for many years with chronic fatigue, immune deficiency resulting in frequent sinus and vaginal yeast infections, painful fibromyalgia symptoms of the back and other muscles, brain fog, and abdominal cramping and bloating. On my recommendation, she did a comprehensive elimination diet. Within the first week of the diet, she felt relief from most of her symptoms, and by the end of the third week of the elimination diet, she said she felt better than she had for many years.

In the reintroduction food-testing phase, Trudy was quickly able to tell that many of her symptoms returned with a vengeance if she consumed wheat (or gluten-containing grains), corn, or tomatoes.

Now that Trudy stays off of these foods, her chronic pain, fatigue, and recurrent infections are dramatically better. She is most thankful for this simple solution to a set of problems that have afflicted and dogged her for most of her adult life. Functional medicine principles and the elimination diet have made a tremendous change in her life.

What You May Expect

The goal of an elimination diet is to clear the body of foods and chemicals you may be allergic or sensitive to. The main rationale behind the diet is that these modifications allow your body's detoxification machinery, which may be overburdened or compromised, to recover and begin to function efficiently again. The dietary changes help your body to eliminate, or clear, various toxins that may have accumulated due to environmental exposure, foods, beverages, drugs, alcohol, or cigarette smoking. These changes also help to reduce inflammation throughout your body.

This is called an *elimination* diet because you completely remove certain foods, and food categories, from your diet. For a period of two to three weeks, you eliminate the foods from your diet that are the most likely culprits. If your symptoms improve during this period, you then carefully add foods back into your diet, one at a time, to see which foods may trigger your symptoms. Throughout the diet, you should make sure to read all labels carefully to find hidden allergens. You should also eat a wide variety of foods and not try to restrict your calorie intake. If you find no improvement within the first three weeks of the diet, either you do not have any food allergies or you may have food allergies but there is yet another factor complicating the picture. There are no magical answers here. This is a journey of self-exploration and discovery.

This process is generally well tolerated and extremely beneficial. In fact, it is one of the best clinical tools available. There is really no typical or normal response. A person's initial response to any new diet is highly variable, and this diet is no exception. This can be attributed to physiological, mental, and biochemical differences among individuals, the degree of exposure to and type of "toxin," and other lifestyle factors. Most often, individuals on the elimination diet report increased energy and mental alertness, decreased muscle or joint pain, and a general sense of improved well-being. However, some people report some initial reactions to the diet, especially in the first week, as their bodies adjust to a different dietary program. Symptoms you may experience in the first week or so include changes in sleep patterns, lightheadedness, headaches, joint or muscle stiffness, and changes in gastrointestinal function. Such symptoms rarely last for more than a few days.

Food Elimination Instructions

The comprehensive elimination diet guidelines in this chapter are intended as a quick overview of the dietary plan. The key is to eat only the foods listed in the "foods to include" column and avoid those foods shown in the "foods to exclude" column. Note that this diet identifies the ten most common allergenic foods: gluten grains, dairy products, eggs, shellfish, corn, peanuts, beef/pork, oranges, soy, and refined sugars. If you have a question about a particular food, check to see if it is on the food list. You should, of course, avoid any listed foods to which you know you are intolerant or allergic. You also may change some of these guidelines based upon your personal health condition and history.

Here are a few tips before you get started.

- The first two to three days are the hardest. It's important to go shopping to get all of the foods you are allowed to have.

- Plan your meals and have a pot of rice available.

- Eat simply. Cook simply. Make a pot of chicken-vegetable-rice soup. Make a large salad. Cook extra chicken. Have prepared food on hand, so you can grab something quickly.

- Eat regular meals.

- You may also want to snack to keep your blood sugar levels normal. Carry food with you when you leave the house, so you will not be tempted to stray off the plan.

- It may be helpful to cook extra chicken, sweet potatoes, rice, and beans, which can be reheated for snacking or another meal.

- Avoid any foods that you know or believe you may be sensitive to, even if they are on the "foods to include" list.

- Try to eat at least three servings of fresh vegetables each day. Choose at least one serving of dark green or orange vegetables (carrots, broccoli, winter squash) and one raw vegetable each day. Vary your selections.

- This is not a weight-loss program. If you need to lose or gain weight, work with your practitioner on a program.

- Buy organic produce when possible. Select fresh foods whenever you can. If possible, choose organically grown fruits and vegetables to eliminate pesticide and chemical residue consumption. Wash fruits and vegetables thoroughly.

- If you are a vegetarian, consume more beans and rice, quinoa, amaranth, teff, millet, and buckwheat instead of meat or fish.

- If you are consuming coffee or other caffeine-containing beverages on a regular basis, it is always wise to slowly reduce your caffeine intake rather than to abruptly stop it; this will prevent caffeine-withdrawal headaches. For instance, try drinking half decaf/half regular coffee for a few days, and then slowly reduce the total amount of coffee.

- Read oil labels. Use only those that are obtained by a cold-press method.

- If you select animal sources of protein, look for free-range or organically raised chicken, turkey, or lamb. Trim visible fat and prepare by broiling, baking, stewing, grilling, or stir-frying. Cold-water fish (salmon, mackerel, and halibut) is another excellent source of protein and the omega-3 essential fatty acids, which are important nutrients in this diet. Fish is used extensively.

- Remember to drink at least two quarts of plain, filtered water each day.

- Strenuous or prolonged exercise may be reduced during some of or for the entire program to allow your body to heal more effectively without the additional burden imposed by exercise. Adequate rest and stress reduction are also important to the success of this program.

Comprehensive Elimination Diet Guidelines

Foods to Include	Foods to Exclude
Fruits: whole fruits, unsweetened, frozen or water packed, canned fruits and diluted juices	Oranges and orange juice
Dairy substitutes: rice milk	Dairy and eggs: milk, cheese, eggs, cottage cheese, cream, yogurt, butter, ice cream, frozen yogurt, nondairy creamers
Nongluten grains and starch: rice (all types), millet, quinoa, amaranth, teff, tapioca, buckwheat, potato flour	Gluten-containing grains: Wheat, corn, barley, spelt, rye, triticale, oat
Animal protein: fresh or water-packed canned fish, wild game, lamb, duck, organic chicken and turkey	Pork, beef/veal, sausage, cold cuts, canned meats, frankfurters, shellfish
Vegetable proteins: split peas, lentils, and legumes (to be included only if you are a vegetarian)	Soybean products: soy sauce, soybean oil in processed foods; tempeh, tofu, soymilk, soy yogurt, textured vegetable protein
Nuts and seeds: Coconut, pine nuts, flaxseed	Peanuts and peanut butter, walnuts, sesame, pumpkin, and sunflower seeds, hazelnuts, pecans, almonds, cashews, nut butters such as almond or tahini
Vegetables: all raw, steamed, sautéed, juiced, or roasted vegetables	Corn, creamed vegetables. (If you have arthritis, avoid nightshades: tomatoes, potatoes, eggplants, peppers, paprika, salsa, chili peppers, cayenne, chili powder.)
Oils and fats: cold pressed olive, ghee	Butter, margarine, shortening, processed oils, salad dressings, mayonnaise, and spreads, flax, safflower, sesame, almond, sunflower, walnut, canola, pumpkin
Drinks: filtered or distilled water, decaffeinated herbal teas, seltzer or mineral water	Alcohol, coffee, and other caffeinated beverages, soda pop or soft drinks
Sweeteners (used sparingly): brown rice syrup, agave nectar, stevia, fruit sweetener, blackstrap molasses	Refined sugar, white/brown sugars, honey, maple syrup, high-fructose corn syrup, evaporated cane juice
Condiments: vinegar, all spices, including salt, pepper, basil, carob, cinnamon, cumin, dill, garlic, ginger, mustard, oregano, parsley, rosemary, tarragon, thyme, turmeric	Chocolate, ketchup, relish, chutney, soy sauce, barbecue sauce, teriyaki, and other condiments

Watch out for the following:

- Baking powder and processed foods may contain cornstarch.

- Many beverages and processed foods contain corn syrup.

- Vinegar in ketchup, mayonnaise, and mustard is usually from wheat or corn.

- Breads advertised as gluten-free may contain oats, spelt, kamut, or rye.

- Many amaranth and millet flake cereals have oats or corn.

- Many canned tunas contain textured vegetable protein, which is from soy; look for low-salt versions which tend to be pure tuna, with no fillers.

Food Reintroduction

Once you have completed two or three weeks of the elimination diet, you can begin to add foods back. Be sure to add foods one at a time, one every two days. Eat the test food at least twice a day and in a fairly large amount. You will want to wait two full days to see if you have a reaction. Assess your response over the next forty-eight to seventy-two hours.

You should keep a journal of all foods eaten and all symptoms that you notice. Often an offending food will provoke symptoms quickly—within ten minutes—or more gradually, up to twelve hours after ingestion. Signs to look for include headache, itching, bloating, nausea, dizziness, fatigue, diarrhea, indigestion, anal itching, feeling sleepy thirty minutes after a meal, flushing, and rapid heartbeat. If you are unsure, take the food back out of your diet for at least one week and try reintroducing it again. Be sure to test foods in a pure form: for example, test milk or cheese or wheat, but not macaroni and cheese that contains milk, cheese, and wheat!

You can use the following chart to document what happens as you reintroduce foods. Clearly mark the day, the food consumed, and your symptoms. You may insert different headings corresponding to whatever signs or symptoms that you may display. Important indicators that must be charted, however, include digestion/bowel function and energy level. If you require more space, you can simply copy this sheet. Again, if you are unsure if you have had a reaction, you can retest the same food by eliminating and reintroducing it once more.

Comprehensive elimination diet adapted from the Institute for Functional Medicine

Day	Food/ Time Eaten	Digestion/ Bowel Function	Joint/ Muscle Aches	Headache/ Pressure	Nasal or Chest Congestion	Kidney- Bladder	Skin Symptoms	Other Symptoms	Energy Level

The Results

By avoiding symptom-provoking foods and taking supportive supplements to restore gut integrity, most food allergies/sensitivities will resolve within four to six months. This means that in most cases, you will be able to once again eat foods that formerly bothered you. In some cases, you will find that the allergy doesn't go away. In this case, either you must wait longer or you may have a fixed allergy that will remain lifelong. After the testing, it would be advisable to return to your health practitioner for a follow-up visit to determine your next steps if you detect significant reactions to any food.

The comprehensive elimination diet described in this chapter will help you determine if you have an allergy or sensitivity to gluten grains, dairy products, eggs, shellfish, peanuts, corn, beef/pork, soy, oranges, or refined sugars. The so-called caveman diet is a simplified but even stricter elimination diet with food intake limited to lamb, rice, pears, and sweet potatoes. You may not ever want to eat any of these again after two to three weeks on the caveman diet.

If you were to eliminate only two things to see if they are the culprits in your condition, they would be wheat and dairy, since these are the most common allergenic foods. You can use the same process as the one described in this chapter, but just eliminate and then reintroduce wheat and dairy. Be careful and watch out for many hidden sources of wheat, gluten, and various dairy-related foods, additives, and so on. Read labels if you are unsure.

THE HIGH-FIBER DIET

Perhaps there is no dietary change you can make that is as simple or important as increasing your fiber intake. Fiber is the part of plants that is either soluble or insoluble in liquid but indigestible. It is made from the cell walls and cellulose of common grains, legumes, fruits, and vegetables. High-fiber diets are excellent for many GI conditions and may reduce the risk or symptoms of not only constipation but also appendicitis, hemorrhoids, hernias, diverticulosis, irritable bowel, colon polyps, and colon cancer. Fiber can act as a prebiotic to support healthy bacteria. Also, by slowing the transit of intestinal contents, fiber reduces cholesterol, slows release of sugar and insulin, and reduces the risk of obesity.

So how much fiber do you need and how do you get it? Recommended levels of fiber are twenty to thirty grams or higher daily, though most American diets contain less than half of this amount. Meat, milk, eggs, and other dairy products contain no fiber. The following table includes some of the best sources of fiber.

Fiber in Foods

Legumes (cooked)	Serving Size	Fiber Content
Black beans	one cup	15 g
Pinto beans	one cup	15 g
Kidney beans	one cup	6 g
Whole Grains and Cereals		
Oatmeal (cooked)	one cup	6 g
Whole grain bread	one slice	3 g
Brown rice (cooked)	one-half cup	2 g
Vegetables		
Broccoli (cooked or raw)	one cup	3 g
Romaine lettuce	one cup	1 g
Spinach	one cup	2 g
Fruits		
Apple (with skin)	medium	4 g
Pear	medium	4 g
Raspberries	one cup	8 g
Nuts and Seeds		
Peanuts	one ounce	2 g
Walnuts	eight whole	2 g
Sunflower seeds	one ounce	2.5 g

This list of high-fiber foods was assembled from a number of different sources. More complete lists are available online. The Mayo Clinic and the U.S. Department of Agriculture both have helpful information (see resources).

Clearly, beans and legumes easily provide the most fiber per serving, followed by whole grains. Selected fruits and vegetables, like raspberries and broccoli, are also especially high in fiber. While you might notice some bloating and gas as you increase the fiber content in your diet, your system should gradually adjust. If you check your stools, the higher the fiber in your diet, the more positive difference you'll notice in terms of bulk and "floaties."

If you follow the recommendations made in the SuperFoods pyramid (see chapter 4) or Mediterranean diet pyramid (see resources), you can quite easily increase your fiber content and your GI health.

DETOXIFICATION PROGRAM

Our environment has become increasingly challenging to our metabolism as we are exposed to more and more chemicals, pesticides, herbicides, air- and water-borne pollutants, hormones, antibiotics, and other toxins. Such exposures can start before birth in the vulnerable prenatal period and continue throughout our lifetimes. Undergoing periodic detoxification through cleansing, diet, supplements, and sauna and steam treatments can help to minimize the impact of these toxins on our genes and other metabolic processes.

A gradual so-called detoxification lifestyle may be more useful than episodic binges of fasting, purging, colonic enemas, and other more extreme measures. By and large, we accumulate these toxins gradually, so it makes sense to try to eliminate them from our lifestyles.

The Detoxifying Lifestyle

The point of any detoxification process is to assist your body's own processes, particularly in the liver and intestinal tract, to function better and to relieve these organs of their overwork. The detoxifying lifestyle method focuses on prevention and reducing toxins through lifestyle changes:

- Reduce exposure in both home and work to toxins through proper filtration and ventilation processes.

- Use organically grown foods as much as possible, and be sure to wash and cleanse foods that you do not peel, so you remove agricultural chemicals.

- Use household cleaning products that decrease impact on the environment.

- Keep abundant house plants to clean indoor air.

- Select fish and seafood that are lower in mercury and other toxins.

- Avoid fatty meats, as toxins are concentrated in fat cells.

- Increase intake of foods known to stimulate detoxification, such as apples, citrus, onions, garlic, soy, broccoli, tea, and various spices and foods rich in calcium and iron.

- Support detoxification systems with foods or supplements rich in antioxidant-containing SuperFoods with B vitamins, vitamin C, vitamin D, magnesium, and selenium.

Following these simple steps will decrease your toxic exposure and load. Such lifestyle measures can not only improve your gut health but also reduce risks of serious illnesses such as cancer and heart disease (Pratt and Kolberg 2009).

A Detox Week

At times, you might feel that a brief, more intense detoxification process is needed. This may be necessary if you have noted problems with intolerance of chemicals, drugs, alcohol, or odors. This is also suggested if you have a history of continuous exposure to pollutants or chemicals in the home or workspace. Some signs or symptoms suggesting toxic overload may include numbness, pain in the muscles or joints, cognitive dysfunction, swelling, and skin rashes (Jones and Quinn 2005).

Here are the basic elements of the program:

1. A brief fast of one to two days limiting yourself to abundant clean water and juices

2. An elemental low-allergenic diet, such as that described in the comprehensive elimination diet above, for five to seven days

3. Regular sauna or steam therapy, three times a week or more on nonfasting days, and shower hydrotherapy daily

4. Selected supplements to help support your body's detoxification processes, including antioxidants (5000 units beta-carotene daily), B vitamins (B50 or B100), vitamin C (2 to 3 g daily), vitamin D (2000 IU daily), selenium (200 to 400 mcg daily), and magnesium (350 to 500 mg in chelated form daily)

At the end of this roughly week-long period, you slowly reintroduce foods; continue hydrotherapy or sauna and supplements for a month to allow your body to continue to adjust to its healthier milieu. Once finished, you should return to the basic principles of prevention discussed in the previous detoxifying lifestyle section (Liska, Lyon, and Jones 2005; Lyon, Bland, and Jones 2005).

CONCLUSION

The diet and detoxification strategies discussed in this chapter can help you identify problem foods, improve bowel function, and reduce the impact of environmental toxins and pollutants on your health. Most people can use these approaches in a home-based and self-directed program. If you have a serious illness, are on multiple medications, or have multiple health conditions, you will want to consult with a nutritionally oriented health care provider before undertaking any of these strategies. If you discover significant health issues related to various foods through using the elimination diet, discuss these with your primary care provider.

CONCLUSION

Tools for life ... this is what *The Healthy Gut Workbook* really is. It provides help and practical advice in solving the kinds of real problems you may experience from time to time or recurrently with your gut health. As you have taken this journey from one end of the digestive tract to the other, I hope you have learned many helpful tips and adopted some good ideas on how to improve your gut health and overall well-being.

You have learned by doing that an emphasis on healthier choices of foods, activities, and mindfulness of your stress can all be essential to protecting your health. Above all, I hope you now recognize how much power you have over your own wellness or illness and claim that power through making informed choices.

To recap, we looked first at the normal processes of healthy gut function and followed this with several chapters about food. These examined the roles of food in our lives, not only nutritionally, but socially, emotionally, and from a preventive-health dimension. I have tried to simplify the often-confusing information about what to eat and what not to eat with the helpful model of well-researched SuperFoods. I emphasized the proven benefits of a Mediterranean diet, and several food pyramids for other cultural and ethnically diverse choices, to guide you in shopping, cooking, and eating. This book also explored the role of inflammation and food allergies and, in all these chapters, helped you take greater notice of your own behaviors and emotions, perhaps as a prelude to adopting a more wellness-promoting lifestyle.

Finally, the book closed with an extensive and holistic review of therapeutic approaches to the healthy gut in conditions of "dis-ease" and when it needs support. The functional-medicine approach of remove, replace, reinoculate, and repair is one of the major approaches that you will find useful, along with the elimination diet in certain circumstances.

In summary, I trust this journey through the gut and its effects on the body has provided you with useful tools for a healthier life for you and your family. Be well, be mindful, eat well, live long, and prosper.

RESOURCES

HEALTHY RECIPES

Bazilian, W., S. Pratt, and K. Matthews. *The Superfoods Rx Diet: Lose Weight with the Power of SuperNutrients*. New York: Rodale Books, 2007.

Bluestein, B., and K. Morrissey. *99 Percent Fat-Free Italian Cooking*. New York: Doubleday, 1999.

Brody, J. *Jane Brody's Good Seafood Book*. New York: W. W. Norton, 1994.

Bugialli, G. *Giuliano Bugialli's Classic Techniques of Italian Cooking*. New York: Simon and Schuster, 1982.

La Cucina Italiana. A magazine dedicated to Italian food and cooking, with recipes and ingredient guides.

LaPuma, J. *Chef MD's Big Book of Culinary Medicine*. New York: Three Rivers Press/Random House, 2008.

Moosewood Collective. *Moosewood Restaurant Low-Fat Favorites: Flavorful Recipes for Healthful Meals*. New York: Clarkson Potter, 1996.

Moosewood Collective. *New Recipes from the Moosewood Restaurant*. Berkeley, CA: Ten Speed Press, 1987.

Passmore, J. *Asia the Beautiful Cookbook*. San Francisco: Collins, 1995.

Pratt, S. *Superfoods Rx: Fourteen Foods That Will Change Your Life*. New York: William Morrow, 2004.

Psilakis, M., and B. Kafka. *How to Roast Lamb: New Greek Classical Cooking*. New York: Little, Brown and Company, 2009.

RECOMMENDED READING

Achterberg, J. *Imagery in Healing*. Boston: New Science Library, 1985.

Benson, H., and E. Stuart. *The Wellness Book: The Comprehensive Guide to Maintaining Health and Treating Stress-Related Illness*. Secaucus, NJ: Birch Lane Press, 1992.

Cordain, L. *The Paleo Diet: Lose Weight and Get Healthy by Eating the Food You Were Designed to Eat*. New York: John Wiley and Sons, 2002.

Davis, M., M. McKay, and E. R. Eshelman. *The Relaxation and Stress Reduction Workbook*. 6th ed. Oakland, CA: New Harbinger, 2008.

Gottschall, E. G. *Breaking the Vicious Cycle: Intestinal Health Through Diet*. Rev. ed. Baltimore: Kirkton Press, 1994.

Karpa, K. D. *Bacteria for Breakfast, Probiotics for Good Health*. Victoria, BC, Canada: Trafford Publishing, 2006.

Nichols, T., and N. Faass. *Optimal Digestive Health: A Complete Guide*. Rochester, Vermont: Healing Arts Press, 2005.

Ornish, D. *Love and Survival*. New York: Harper Collins, 1998.

Pratt, S., and K. Matthews. *SuperFoods HealthStyle: Proven Strategies for Lifelong Health*. New York: William Morrow, 2006.

Pratt, S., and S. Kolberg. *SuperHealth: 6 Simple Steps, 6 Easy Weeks, 1 Longer, Healthier Life*. New York: Dutton, 2008.

Rakel, D. *Integrative Medicine*. 2nd ed. Philadelphia: Saunders, 2007.

Scala, J. *The New Eating Right for a Bad Gut: The Complete Nutritional Guide to Ileitis, Colitis, Crohn's Disease, and Inflammatory Bowel Disease*. New York: Plume, 2000.

Sears, B. 2004. *The Anti-Inflammation Zone: Reversing the Silent Epidemic That's Destroying Our Health*. New York: Harper Collins.

Sierpina, V. *Integrative Health Care: Alternative and Complementary Therapies for the Whole Person*. Philadelphia: FA Davis, 2001.

Sierpina, V., and C. Gustafson, Z. Ren, B. MacEoin, G. Espinosa, and D. Kiefer. *1000 Cures for 200 Ailments: Integrated Alternative and Conventional Treatments for Most Common Illnesses*. New York: Harper Collins, 2007.

Simonton, O. *Getting Well Again*. New York: Bantam, 1980.

Tyler, V. *Herbs of Choice: The Therapeutic Use of Phytomedicinals*. New York: Pharmaceutical Products Press, 1994.

FOOD PYRAMIDS

Asian Diet Pyramid. The traditional Asian diet as a model for healthy eating. Includes an exercise at the base, from Oldways. http://www.oldwayspt.org/asian-diet-pyramid.

Healing Foods Pyramid. Gives daily, weekly, and optional foods (including dark chocolate) and uses adequate water intake as a base, from the University of Michigan Department of Integrative Medicine. http://med.umich.edu/umim/food-pyramid/healing_foods_pyramid.jpg.

Latin American Diet Pyramid. Guide to a healthy and traditional Latin American diet, from Oldways. http://www.oldwayspt.org/latino-diet-pyramid.

Mediterranean Diet Pyramid. The Mediterranean diet has been shown in clinical trials to be easier to continue long term with significant improvement in heart health over the standard cardiac diet. This version includes an exercise at the base, from Oldways. http://www.oldwayspt.org/mediterranean-diet-pyramid.

MyPyramid Food Guidance System. Dietary recommendations from the United States Department of Agriculture. Also available in Spanish. http://www.mypyramid.gov/.

Soul Food Pyramid. Based on the traditional African-American diet, including a recipe for orange-honey acorn squash, from the Southeastern Michigan Dietetic Association. http://semda.org/info/pyramid.asp?ID=7.

Vegan Food Pyramid. Dietary recommendations for vegans from Wikimedia Commons. http://en.wikipedia.org/wiki/File:Vegan_food_pyramid.svg.

Vegetarian Diet Pyramid. A healthy traditional vegetarian eating plan, including dairy and eggs, from Oldways. http://www.oldwayspt.org/vegetarian-diet-pyramid.

ONLINE RESOURCES

Holmes and Rahe Stress Scale. A useful tool for measuring your current stress levels, based on recent stress factors in your life. http://en.wikipedia.org/wiki/Holmes_and_Rahe_stress_scale.

International Foundation for Functional Gastrointestinal Disorders. A site for support and information on reflux disease. http://aboutgerd.org/.

Mayo Foundation for Medical Education and Research. Mayo Clinic information and tools for healthy living. Great information on fiber and multiple other topics related to health. The Mayo Clinic has a useful list of high-fiber foods on its website: http://mayoclinic.com/health /high-fiber-foods/NU00582.

National Center for Chronic Disease Prevention and Health Promotion. Helpful information on current fitness and exercise recommendations. http://cdc.gov/physicalacticity/everyone /guidelines/.

National Digestive Diseases Information Clearinghouse. An excellent general resource for all digestive health information. http://digestive.niddk.nih.gov/.

National Foundation for Celiac Awareness. A support group and information site for those afflicted with celiac disease and gluten sensitivity. http://www.celiaccentral.org.

North American Society for Pediatric Gastroenterology, Hepatology, and Nutrition. Dedicated to pediatric gut problems. http://naspghan.org/.

Pediatric/Adolescent Gastroesophageal Reflux Association (PAGER). Devoted to pediatric GERD. http://reflux.org/.

U.S. Department of Agriculture National Agricultural Library Food and Nutrition Information Center. Includes useful information about the health benefits of dietary fiber and a vast array of other nutritional advice. Or go to http://fnic.nal.usda.gov, select "Consumers" from the dropdown list on the left, then click on "Eating for Health" in the Consumer Corner box and "Fiber" from the expanded list."

WebMD, LLC. WebMD: Better information. Better Health. Up-to-date, user-friendly information on general health topics, including gut health. http://www.webmd.com.

Wellness Inventory: Whole Person Assessment Program for physical, spiritual, and emotional wellness. At HealthWorld Online. An online instrument to help you assess and plan for improved health and well-being. http://www.wellpeople.com/index_wp.asp?UID=&Id=.

REFERENCES

Acosta, J. A., M. L. Grebenc, R. C. Doberneck, J. D. McCarthy, and D. E. Fry. 1992. Colonic diverticular disease in patients forty years old or younger. *American Surgeon* 58 (10): 605–7.

Ahmad, N., and H. Mukhtar. 1999. Green tea polyphenols and cancer: Biologic mechanisms and practical implications. *Nutrition Reviews* 57 (3): 78–83.

Albanes, D., O. Heinonen, P. Taylor, J. Virtamo, B. Edwards, M. Rautalahti, et al. 1996. Alpha-tocopherol and beta carotene supplements and lung cancer incidence in the alpha-tocopherol, beta-carotene cancer prevention study: Effects of base-line characteristics and study compliance. *Journal of the National Cancer Institute* 88: 1560–70.

Albert, C., J. Gaziano, W. Willett, and J. Manson. 2002. Nut consumption and decreased risk of sudden cardiac death in the Physicians' Health Study. *Archives of Internal Medicine* 162 (12): 1382–87.

Albert, C., C. Hennekens, C. O'Donnell, U. Ajani, V. Carey, W. Willett, J. Ruskin, and J. Manson. 1998. Fish consumption and risk of sudden cardiac death. *Journal of the American Medical Association* 279 (1): 23–28.

Aldoori, W. H., E. L. Giovannucci, E. B. Rimm, A. Ascherio, M. J. Stampfer, G. A. Colditz, A. L. Wing, D. V. Trichopoulos, and W. C. Willett. 1995. Prospective study of physical activity and the risk of symptomatic diverticular disease in men. *Gut* 36 (2): 276–82.

Aldoori, W. H., E. L. Giovannucci, E. B. Rimm, A. L. Wing, D. V. Trichopoulos, and W. C. Willett. 1994. A prospective study of diet and the risk of symptomatic diverticular disease in men. *American Journal of Clinical Nutrition* 60 (5): 757–64.

Allen, S., B. Okoko, E. Martinez, G. Gregorio, and L. Dans. 2004. Probiotics for treating infectious diarrhoea. *Cochrane Database Systematic Reviews* 2: CD003048.

Alonso-Coello, P., E. Mills, D. Heels-Ansdell, M. Lopez-Yarto, Q. Zhou, J. F. Johanson, and G. Guyatt. 2006. Fiber for the treatment of hemorrhoids complications: A systematic review and meta-analysis. *American Journal of Gastroenterology* 101 (1): 181–88.

Anderson, J, and N. Gustafson. 1988. Hypocholesterolemic effects of oat and bean products. *American Journal of Clinical Nutrition* 48 (3): 749–53.

Andreone, P., A. Gramonzi, and M. Bernardi. 1998. Vitamin E for chronic hepatitis B. *Annals of Internal Medicine* 128 (2): 156–57.

Ascherio, A., E. Rimm, M. Hernan, E. Giovannucci, I. Kawachi, M. Stampfer, and W. Willett. 1999. Relation of consumption of vitamin E, vitamin C, and carotenoids to risk for stroke among men in the United States. *Annals of Internal Medicine* 130 (12): 963–70.

Aslan, A., and G. Triadafilopoulos. 1992. Fish oil fatty acid supplementation in active ulcerative colitis: A double-blind, placebo-controlled, crossover study. *American Journal of Gastroenterology* 87 (4): 432–37.

Bazilian, W., and S. Pratt. 2008. *The Superfoods Rx Diet: Lose Weight with the Power of Supernutrients.* New York: Rodale.

Belluzzi, A., C. Brignola, M. Campieri, A. Pera, S. Boschi, and M. Miglioli. 1996. Effect of an enteric-coated fish-oil preparation on relapses in Crohn's disease. *New England Journal of Medicine* 334 (24): 1557–60.

Ben-Arye, E., E. Goldin, D. Wengrower, A. Stamper, R. Kohn, and E. Berry. 2002. Wheat grass juice in the treatment of active distal ulcerative colitis: A randomized double-blind placebo-controlled trial. *Scandinavian Journal of Gastroenterology* 37 (4): 444–49.

Bengmark, S. 1998. Ecological control of the gastrointestinal tract. The role of probiotic flora. *Gut* 42 (1): 2–7.

Bennet, J., and M. Brinkman. 1989. Treatment of ulcerative colitis by implantation of normal colonic flora. *Lancet* 1 (8630): 164.

Benson, H. 1975. *The Relaxation Response.* New York: William Morrow.

———. 1984. *Beyond the Relaxation Response.* New York: Times Books.

Benson, H., and E. Stuart. 1992. *The Wellness Book: The Comprehensive Guide to Maintaining Health and Treating Stress-Related Illness.* Secaucus, NJ: Birch Lane Press.

Bensoussan, A., N. J. Talley, M. Hing, R. Menzies, A. Guo, and M. Ngu. 1998. Treatment of irritable bowel syndrome with Chinese herbal medicine: A randomized controlled trial. *Journal of the American Medical Association* 280 (18): 1585–89.

Bhatia, V., and R. K. Tandon. 2005. Stress and the gastrointestinal tract. *Journal of Gastroenterology and Hepatology* 20 (3): 332–39.

Bhatnagar, D., and P. Durrington. 2003. Omega-3 fatty acids: Their role in the prevention and treatment of atherosclerosis related risk factors and complications. *International Journal of Clinical Practice* 57 (4): 301–14.

Bohm, S. K., and W. Kruis. 2006. Probiotics: Do they help to control intestinal inflammation? *Annals of the New York Academy of Sciences* 1072: 339–50.

Bohmer, C. J., and H. A. Tuynman. 1996. The clinical relevance of lactose malabsorption in irritable bowel syndrome. *European Journal of Gastroenterology and Hepatology* 8 (10): 1013–16.

Borody, T., E. Warren, S. Leis, R. Surace, and O. Ashman. 2003. Treatment of ulcerative colitis using fecal bacteriotherapy. *Journal of Clinical Gastroenterology* 37 (1): 42–47.

Bowen, P., V. Garg, M. Stacewicz-Sapuntzakis, L. Yelton, and R. Schreiner. 1993. Variability of serum carotenoids in response to controlled diets containing six servings of fruits and vegetables per day. *Annals of the New York Academy of Sciences* 691: 241–43.

Brenner, D. M., M. J. Moeller, W. D. Chey, and P. S. Schoenfeld. 2009. The utility of probiotics in the treatment of irritable bowel syndrome: A systematic review. *American Journal of Gastroenterology* 104 (4): 1033–49.

Brogden, R. N., T. M. Speight, and G. S. Avery. 1974. Deglycyrrhizinised liquorice: A report of its pharmacological properties and therapeutic efficacy in peptic ulcer. *Drugs* 8 (5): 330–39.

Brown, L., B. Rosner, W. Willett, and F. Sacks. 1999. Cholesterol-lowering effects of dietary fiber: A meta-analysis. *American Journal of Clinical Nutrition* 69 (1): 30–42.

Candy, S., G. Borok, J. P. Wright, V. Boniface, and R. Goodman. 1995. The value of an elimination diet in the management of patients with ulcerative colitis. *South African Medical Journal Suid-Afrikaanse Tydskrif Vir Geneeskunde* 85 (11): 1176–79.

Cao, G., E. Sofic, and R. Prior. 1996. Antioxidant capacity of tea and common vegetables. *Journal of Agricultural and Food Chemistry* 44 (1): 3426–31.

Cao, G., R. Russell, D. Lischner, and R. Prior. 1998. Serum antioxidant capacity is increased by consumption of strawberries, spinach, red wine, or vitamin C in elderly women. *The Journal of Nutrition* 128 (12): 2383–90.

Centers for Disease Control and Prevention. 2008. *How much physical activity do adults need?* http://www.cdc.gov/physicalactivity/everyone/guidelines/adults.html (accessed May 15, 2010).

Cheney, G. 1949. Rapid healing of peptic ulcers in patients receiving fresh cabbage juice. *California Medicine* 70 (1): 10–15.

Chiorean, M. V., G. R. Locke, III, A. R. Zinsmeister, C. D. Schleck, and L. J. Melton, III. 2002. Changing rates of *Helicobacter pylori* testing and treatment in patients with peptic ulcer disease. *American Journal of Gastroenterology* 97: 3015–22.

Chitkara, D. K., A. J. Bredenoord, M. J. Rucker, and N. J. Talley. 2005. Aerophagia in adults: A comparison with functional dyspepsia. *Alimentary Pharmacology and Therapeutics* 22 (9): 855–58.

Clark, L., G. Combs Jr., B. Turnbull, E. Slate, D. Chalker, J. Chow, et al. 1996. Effects of selenium supplementation for cancer prevention in patients with carcinoma of the skin: A randomized controlled trial. Nutritional Prevention of Cancer Study Group. *Journal of the American Medical Association* 276 (24): 1957–63.

Cleveland, L., A. Moshfegh, A. Albertson, and J. Goldman. 2000. Dietary intake of whole grains. *Journal of the American College of Nutrition* 19 (3): S331–38.

Cohen, J., A. Kristal, and J. Stanford. 2000. Fruit and vegetable intakes and prostate cancer risk. *Journal of the National Cancer Institute* 92 (1): 61–68.

Colditz, G., L. Branch, R. Lipnick, W. Willett, B. Rosner, B. Posner, and C. Hennekens. 1985. Increased green and yellow vegetable intake and lowered cancer deaths in an elderly population. *American Journal of Clinical Nutrition* 41 (1): 32–36.

Colomer, R., R. Lupu, A. Papadimitropoulou, L. Vellon, A. Vazquez-Martin, J. Brunet, A. Fernandez-Gutierrez, A. Segura-Carretero, and J. A. Menendez. 2008. Giacomo Castelvetro's salads. Anti-HER2 oncogene nutraceuticals since the seventeenth century? *Clinical and Translational Oncology: Official Publication of the Federation of Spanish Oncology Societies and of the National Cancer Institute of Mexico* 10 (1): 30–34.

Commenges, D., V. Scotet, S. Renaud, H. Jacqmin-Gadda, P. Barberger-Gateau, and J. Dartigues. 2000. Intake of flavonoids and risk of dementia. *European Journal of Epidemiology* 16 (4): 357–63.

Crowell, P. 1999. Prevention and therapy of cancer by dietary monoterpenes. *The Journal of Nutrition* 129 (3): 775S–78S.

Dancey, C. P., M. Taghavi, and R. J. Fox. 1998. The relationship between daily stress and symptoms of irritable bowel: A time-series approach. *Journal of Psychosomatic Research* 44 (5): 537–45.

Davis, M., M. McKay, and E. R. Eshelman. 2008. *The Relaxation and Stress Reduction Workbook*. 6th ed. Oakland, CA: New Harbinger.

de Lorgeril, M., S. Renaud, N. Mamelle, P. Salen, J. Martin, I. Monjaud, J. Guidollet, P. Touboul, and J. Delaye. 1994. Mediterranean alpha-linolenic acid-rich diet in secondary prevention of coronary heart disease. *Lancet* 343 (8911): 1454–59.

De Palma, G., I. Nadal, M. Collado, and Y. Sanz. 2009. Effects of a gluten-free diet on gut microbiota and immune function in healthy adult human subjects. *British Journal of Nutrition* 102 (8): 1154–60.

Dichi, I., P. Frenhane, J. B. Dichi, C. R. Correa, A. Y. Angeleli, M. H. Bicudo, M. A. Rodrigues, C. R. Victoria, and R. C. Burini. 2000. Comparison of omega-3 fatty acids and sulfasalazine in ulcerative colitis. *Nutrition* 16 (2): 87–90.

Duffy, S., J. Keaney Jr., M. Holbrook, N. Gokce, P. Swerdloff, B. Frei, and J. Vita. 2001. Short- and long-term black tea consumption reverses endothelial dysfunction in patients with coronary artery disease. *Circulation* 104 (2): 151–56.

Eaton, S., and M. Konner. 1985. Paleolithic nutrition: Consideration of its nature and current implications. *New England Journal of Medicine* 312 (5): 283–89.

Epocrates, Inc. 2010. http://www.epocrates.com (accessed May 14, 2010).

Etzioni, D. A., T. M. Mack, R. W. Beart Jr., and A. M. Kaiser. 2009. Diverticulitis in the United States: 1998-2005: Changing patterns of disease and treatment. *Annals of Surgery* 249 (2): 210–17.

Fasano, A. 2009. Surprises from celiac disease. *Scientific American* 301 (2): 54–61.

Fujimori, S., K. Gudis, K. Mitsui, T. Seo, M. Yonezawa, S. Tanaka, A. Tatsuguchi, and C. Sakamoto. 2009. A randomized controlled trial on the efficacy of synbiotic versus probiotic or prebiotic treatment to improve the quality of life in patients with ulcerative colitis. *Nutrition* 25 (5): 520–25.

Ganiats, T. G., W. A. Norcross, A. L. Halverson, P. A. Burford, and L. A. Palinkas. 1994. Does Beano prevent gas? A double-blind crossover study of oral alpha-galactosidase to treat dietary oligosaccharide intolerance. *Journal of Family Practice* 39 (5): 441–45.

Geleijnse, J., L. Launer, D. Van der Kuip, A. Hofman, and J. Witteman. 2002. Inverse association of tea and flavonoid intakes with incident myocardial infarction: The Rotterdam study. *American Journal of Clinical Nutrition* 75 (5): 880–86.

Giovannucci, E. 1999. Tomatoes, tomato-based products, lycopene, and cancer: Review of the epidemiologic literature. *Journal of the National Cancer Institute* 91 (4): 317–31.

Goodwin, J. S., and J. M. Goodwin. 1984. The tomato effect. Rejection of highly efficacious therapies. *Journal of the American Medical Association* 251 (18): 2387–90.

Graf, E., and J. Eaton. 1993. Suppression of colonic cancer by dietary phytic acid. *Nutrition and Cancer* 19 (1): 11–19.

Grodstein, F., G. A. Colditz, D. J. Hunter, J. E. Manson, W. C. Willett, and M. J. Stampfer. 1994. A prospective study of symptomatic gallstones in women: Relation with oral contraceptives and other risk factors. *Obstetrics and Gynecology* 84 (2): 207–14.

Gupta, I., A. Parihar, P. Malhotra, G. B. Singh, R. Ludtke, H. Safayhi, and H. P. Ammon. 1997. Effects of Boswellia serrata gum resin in patients with ulcerative colitis. *European Journal of Medical Research* 2 (1): 37–43.

Guralnik, J. M., and G. A. Kaplan. 1989. Predictors of healthy aging: Prospective evidence from the Alameda County study. *American Journal of Public Health* 79 (6): 703–8.

Hanai, H., T. Iida, K. Takeuchi, F. Watanabe, Y. Maruyama, A. Andoh, et al. 2006. Curcumin maintenance therapy for ulcerative colitis: Randomized, multicenter, double-blind, placebo-controlled trial. *Clinical Gastroenterology and Hepatology* 4 (12): 1502–6.

Hegarty, V., H. May, and K. Khaw. 2000. Tea drinking and bone mineral density in older women. *American Journal of Clinical Nutrition* 71 (4): 1003–7.

Heilbrun, L., A. Nomura, and G. Stemmermann. 1986. Black tea consumption and cancer risk: A prospective study. *British Journal of Cancer* 54 (4): 677–83.

Heymen, S., K. R. Jones, Y. Scarlett, and W. E. Whitehead. 2003. Biofeedback treatment of constipation: A critical review. *Diseases of the Colon and Rectum* 46 (9): 1208–17.

Hijazi, Z., A Molla, H. Al-Habashi, W. Muawad, A. Molla, and P. Sharma. 2004. Intestinal permeability is increased in bronchial asthma. *Archives of Disease in Childhood* 89 (3): 227–29.

Hill, A. M., J. D. Buckley, K. J. Murphy, and P. R. C. Howe. 2007. Combining fish-oil supplements with regular aerobic exercise improves body composition and cardiovascular disease risk factors. *American Journal of Clinical Nutrition* 85 (5): 1267–74.

Holman, H. 2004. Chronic disease: The need for a new clinical education. *Journal of the American Medical Association* 292 (9): 1057–59.

Holmes, T. H., and R. H. Rahe. 1967. The social readjustment rating scale. *Journal of Psychosomatic Research* 11 (2): 213–18.

Hujoel, P. P., M. Drangsholt, C. Spiekerman, and T. A. DeRouen. 2000. Periodontal disease and coronary heart disease risk. *Journal of the American Medical Association* 284:1406–10.

Huwez, F. U., D. Thirlwell, A. Cockayne, and D. A. Ala'Aldeen. 1998. Mastic gum kills *Helicobacter pylori*. *New England Journal of Medicine* 339 (26): 1946–48.

Jenab, M., P. Ferrari, N. Slimani, T. Norat, C. Casagrande, K. Overad, et al. 2004. Association of nut and seed intake with colorectal cancer risk in the European prospective investigation into cancer and nutrition. 2004. *Cancer Epidemiology, Biomarkers and Prevention* 13 (10): 1595–603.

Jiang, R., J. Manson, M. Stampfer, S. Liu, W. Willett, and F. Hu. 2002. Nut and peanut butter consumption and risk of type 2 diabetes in women. *Journal of the American Medical Association* 288 (20): 2554–60.

Johanson, J. F., and A. Sonnenberg. 1990. The prevalence of hemorrhoids and chronic constipation. An epidemiologic study. *Gastroenterology* 98 (2): 380–86.

———. 1994. Constipation is not a risk factor for hemorrhoids: A case-control study of potential etiological agents. *American Journal of Gastroenterology* 89 (11): 1981–86.

John, J., S. Ziebland, P. Yudkin, L. Roe, H. Neil, and Oxford Fruit and Vegetable Study Group. 2002. Effects of fruit and vegetable consumption on plasma antioxidant concentrations and blood pressure: A randomized controlled trial. *Lancet* 359 (9322): 1969–74.

Johnston, C. S. 2005. Strategies for healthy weight loss: From vitamin C to the glycemic response. *Journal of the American College of Nutrition* 24 (3): 158–65.

Jones, D., and S. Quinn. 2005. *Textbook of Functional Medicine.* Gig Harbor, WA: The Institute for Functional Medicine.

Kabat-Zinn, J. 1990. *Full Catastrophe Living: Using the Wisdom of Your Body and Mind to Face Stress, Pain and Illness.* New York: Delacorte Press.

Kajander, K., E. Myllyluoma, M. Rajilic-Stojanovic, S. Kyronpalo, M. Rasmussen, S. Jarvenpaa, E. G. Zoetendal, W. M. de Vos, H. Vapaatalo, and R. Korpela. 2008. Clinical trial: Multispecies probiotic supplementation alleviates the symptoms of irritable bowel syndrome and stabilizes intestinal microbiota. *Alimentary Pharmacology and Therapeutics* 27 (1): 48–57.

Kalliomaki, M., S. Salminen, T. Poussa, and E. Isolauri. 2007. Probiotics during the first seven years of life: A cumulative risk reduction of eczema in a randomized, placebo-controlled trial. *The Journal of Allergy and Clinical Immunology* 119 (4): 1019–21.

Kalliomaki, M., S. Salminen, T. Poussa, H. Arvilommi, and E. Isolauri. 2003. Probiotics and prevention of atopic disease: Four-year follow-up of a randomised placebo-controlled trial. *Lancet* 361 (9372): 1869–71.

Kamiji, M. M., and R. B. de Oliveira. 2005. Nonantibiotic therapies for *Helicobacter pylori* infection. *European Journal of Gastroenterology and Hepatology* 17 (9): 973–81.

Kaptchuk, T., J. Kelley, L. Conboy, R. Davis, C. Kerr, E. Jacobson, et al. 2008. Components of placebo effect: Randomised controlled trial in patients with irritable bowel syndrome. *British Medical Journal* 336 (7651): 999–1003.

King, T. S., M. Elia, and J. O. Hunter. 1998. Abnormal colonic fermentation in irritable bowel syndrome. *Lancet* 352 (9135): 1187–89.

Kirk, G. R., J. S. White, L. McKie, M. Stevenson, I. Young, W. D. Clements, and B. J. Rowlands. 2006. Combined antioxidant therapy reduces pain and improves quality of life in chronic pancreatitis. *Journal of Gastrointestinal Surgery* 10 (4): 499–503.

Kligler, B., and A. Cohrssen. 2008. Probiotics. *American Family Physician* 79 (9): 1073–78.

Kockar, C., M. Ozturk, and N. Bavbek. 2001. *Helicobacter pylori* eradication with beta carotene, ascorbic acid and allicin. *Acta Medica (Hradec Kralove)* 44 (3): 97–100.

Krinsky, N. 1998. The antioxidant and biological properties of the carotenoids. *Annals of the New York Academy of Sciences* 854: 443–47.

Kris-Etherton, P., W. Harris, L. Appel, and American Heart Association Nutrition Committee. 2002. Fish consumption, fish oil, omega-3 fatty acids and cardiovascular disease. *Circulation* 106 (21): 2747–57.

Kris-Etherton, P., W. Harris, and L. Appel for the American Hearth Association Nutrition Committee. 2003. Omega-3 fatty acids and cardiovascular disease: New recommendations from the American Heart Association. *Arteriosclerosis, Thrombosis, and Vascular Biology* 23: 151–52.

Kushi, L., K. Meyer, and D. Jacobs, Jr. 1999. Cereals, legumes, and chronic disease risk reduction: Evidence from epidemiologic studies. *American Journal of Clinical Nutrition* 70 (3): S451–58.

Lack, G. 2008. Clinical practice. Food allergy. *New England Journal of Medicine* 359 (12): 1252–60.

Lackner, J. M., J. Jaccard, S. S. Krasner, L. A. Katz, G. D. Gudleski, and E. B. Blanchard. 2007. How does cognitive behavior therapy for irritable bowel syndrome work? A mediational analysis of a randomized clinical trial. *Gastroenterology* 133 (2): 433–34.

Laheij, R. J., M. C. Sturkenboom, R. J. Hassing, J. Dieleman, B. H. Stricker, and J. B. Jansen. 2004. Risk of community-acquired pneumonia and use of gastric acid-suppressive drugs. *Journal of the American Medical Association* 292 (16): 1955–60.

Langmead, L., R. M. Feakins, S. Goldthorpe, H. Holt, E. Tsironi, A. De Silva, D. P. Jewell, and D. S. Rampton. 2004. Randomized, double-blind, placebo-controlled trial of oral aloe vera gel for active ulcerative colitis. *Alimentary Pharmacology and Therapeutics* 19 (7): 739–47.

Lasser, R. B., J. H. Bond, and M. D. Levitt. 1975. The role of intestinal gas in functional abdominal pain. *New England Journal of Medicine* 293 (11): 524–26.

Leitzmann, M. F., W. C. Willett, E. B. Rimm, M. J. Stampfer, D. Spiegelman, G. A. Colditz, and E. Giovannucci. 1999. A prospective study of coffee consumption and the risk of symptomatic gallstone disease in men. *Journal of the American Medical Association* 281 (22): 2106–12.

Lemieux, I., A. Pascot, D. Prud'homme, N. Alméras, P. Bogaty, A. Nadeau, J. Bergeron, and J. P. Després. 2001. Elevated C-reactive protein: Another component of the atherothrombotic profile of abdominal obesity. *Arteriosclerosis, Thrombosis, and Vascular Biology* 21: 961–67.

Levenstein, S., S. Ackerman, J. K. Kiecolt-Glaser, and A. Dubois. 1999. Stress and peptic ulcer disease. *Journal of the American Medical Association* 281 (1): 10–11.

Liska, D., M. Lyon, and D. Jones. 2005. Detoxification and biotransformation imbalances. In *Textbook of Functional Medicine*, edited by D. Jones and S. Quinn. Gig Harbor, WA: The Institute for Functional Medicine.

Litonjua, A. A., D. K. Milton, J. C. Celedon, L. Ryan, S. T. Weiss, and D. R. Gold. 2002. A longitudinal analysis of wheezing in young children: The independent effects of early life exposure to house dust endotoxin, allergens, and pets. *Journal of Allergy and Clinical Immunology* 110 (5): 736–42.

Liu, J. P., M. Yang, Y. X. Liu, M. L. Wei, and S. Grimsgaard. 2006. Herbal medicines for treatment of irritable bowel syndrome. *Cochrane Database of Systematic Reviews* (1): CD004116.

Liu, L., S. Zhao, M. Gao, Q. Zhou, Y. Li, and B. Xia. 2002. Vitamin C preserves endothelial function in patients with coronary heart disease after a high-fat meal. *Clinical Cardiology* 25 (5): 219–24.

Liu, S., J. Manson, J. Buring, M. Stampfer, W. Willett, and P. Ridker. 2002. Relation between a diet with a high glycemic load and plasma concentrations of high-sensitivity C-reactive protein in middle-aged women. *American Journal of Clinical Nutrition* 75 (3): 492–8.

Loguercio, C., and A. Federico. 2003. Oxidative stress in viral and alcoholic hepatitis. *Free Radical Biology and Medicine* 34 (1): 1–10.

Lovejoy, J., M. Most, M. Lefevre, F. Greenway, and J. Rood. 2002. Effect of diets enriched in almonds on insulin action and serum lipids in adults with normal glucose tolerance or type 2 diabetes. *American Journal of Clinical Nutrition* 76 (5): 1000–1006.

Lyon, M., J. Bland, and D. Jones. 2005. Clinical approaches to detoxification and biotransformation. In *Textbook of Functional Medicine*, edited by D. Jones and S. Quinn. Gig Harbor, WA: The Institute for Functional Medicine.

Maclure, K. M., K. C. Hayes, G. A. Colditz, M. J. Stampfer, F. E. Speizer, and W. C. Willett. 1989. Weight, diet, and the risk of symptomatic gallstones in middle-aged women. *New England Journal of Medicine* 321 (9): 563–69.

Mallon, P., D. McKay, S. Kirk, and K. Gardiner. 2007. Probiotics for induction of remission in ulcerative colitis. *Cochrane Database of Systematic Reviews* (4): CD005573.

Matsui, E. C., R. A. Wood, C. Rand, S. Kanchanaraksa, L. Swartz, and P. A. Eggleston. 2004. Mouse allergen exposure and mouse skin test sensitivity in suburban, middle-class children with asthma. *Journal of Allergy and Clinical Immunology* 113 (5): 910–15.

McKay, D. L., and J. B. Blumberg. 2002. The role of tea in human health: An update. *Journal of the American College of Nutrition* 21 (1): 1–13.

Messina, M., V. Persky, K. Setchell, and S. Barnes. 1994. Soy intake and cancer risk: A review of the in vitro and in vivo data. *Nutrition and Cancer* 21 (2): 113–31.

Michaud, D., Y. Liu, M. Meyer, E. Giovannucci, and K. Joshipura. 2008. Periodontal disease, tooth loss, and cancer risk in male health professionals: A prospective cohort study. *Lancet Oncology* 9 (6): 550–58.

Misciagna, G., S. Centonze, C. Leoci, V. Guerra, A. M. Cisternino, R. Ceo, and M. Trevisan. 1999. Diet, physical activity, and gallstones: A population-based, case-control study in southern Italy. *American Journal of Clinical Nutrition* 69 (1): 120–26.

Misra, M. C., and R. Parshad. 2000. Randomized clinical trial of micronized flavonoids in the early control of bleeding from acute internal hemorrhoids. *British Journal of Surgery* 87 (7): 868–72.

Morris, M. C., D. A. Evans, C. C. Tangney, J. L. Bienias, and R. S. Wilson. 2006. Associations of vegetable and fruit consumption with age-related cognitive change. *Neurology* 67: 1370–76.

Mossner, J. 1993. Is there a place for pancreatic enzymes in the treatment of pain in chronic pancreatitis? *Digestion* 54 (Suppl. 2): 35–39.

Nakamura, R., G. Littarru, K. Folkers, and E. Wilkinson. 1973. Deficiency of coenzyme Q in gingiva of patients with periodontal disease. *International Journal for Vitamin and Nutrition Research* 43 (1): 84–92.

Nestle, M. 1998. Broccoli sprouts in cancer prevention. *Nutrition Reviews* 56 (4): 127–30.

Pack, A. 1984. Folate mouthwash: Effects on established gingivitis in periodontal patients. *Journal of Clinical Periodontology* 11 (9): 619–28.

Peters, H. P., W. R. De Vries, G. P. Vanberge-Henegouwen, and L. M. Akkermans. 2001. Potential benefits and hazards of physical activity and exercise on the gastrointestinal tract. *Gut* 48 (3): 435–39.

Physicians' Desk Reference. 2009. *Physicians' Desk Reference.* 63rd edition. Montvale, NJ: Thomson PDR.

Pischon, N., N. Heng, J. P. Bernimoulin, B. M. Kleber, N. Willich, and T. Pischon. 2007. Obesity, inflammation, and periodontal disease. *Journal of Dental Research* 86: 400–409.

Pischon, T., S. E. Hankinson, G. S. Hotamisligil, N. Rifai, W. C. Willett, and E. B. Rimm. 2003. Habitual dietary intake of n-3 and n-6 fatty acids in relation to inflammatory markers among U.S. men and women. *Circulation* 108 (2): 155–60.

Pittler, M. H., and E. Ernst. 1998. Peppermint oil for irritable bowel syndrome: A critical review and metaanalysis. *American Journal of Gastroenterology* 93 (7): 1131–35.

Pollan, M. 2008. *In Defense of Food: An Eater's Manifesto.* New York: Penguin Press.

Potter, T., C. Ellis, and M. Levitt. 1985. Activated charcoal: In vivo and in vitro studies of effect on gas formation. *Gastroenterology* 88 (3): 620–24.

Pratt, S. 2004. *Superfoods Rx: Fourteen Foods That Will Change Your Life.* New York: William Morrow.

Pratt, S., and K. Matthews. 2005. *Superfoods Healthstyle: Proven Strategies for Lifelong Health.* New York: Harper Collins.

Pratt, S., and S. Kolberg. 2009. *Superhealth: Six Simple Steps, Six Easy Weeks, One Longer, Healthier Life.* New York: Dutton.

Preidis, G. A., and J. Versalovic. 2009. Targeting the human microbiome with antibiotics, probiotics, and prebiotics: Gastroenterology enters the metagenomics era. *Gastroenterology* 136 (6): 2015–31.

Rajaram, S., and J. Sabaté. 2006. Nuts, body weight, and insulin resistance. *British Journal of Nutrition* 96: S79–86.

Rakel, D. P., and A. Rindfleisch. 2005. Inflammation: Nutritional, botanical, and mind-body influences. *Southern Medical Journal* 98 (3): 303–10.

Robertson, D. J., H. Larsson, S. Friis, L. Pedersen, J. A. Baron, and H. T. Sorensen. 2007. Proton pump inhibitor use and risk of colorectal cancer: A population-based, case-control study. *Gastroenterology* 133 (3): 755–60.

Rolfe, R. D. 2000. The role of probiotic cultures in the control of gastrointestinal health. *Journal of Nutrition* 130: S396–402.

Rolfe, V. E., P. J. Fortun, C. J. Hawkey, and F. Bath-Hextall. 2006. Probiotics for maintenance of remission in Crohn's disease. *Cochrane Database of Systematic Reviews* (4): CD004826.

Ruemmele, F., D. Bier, P. Marteau, G. Rechkemmer, R. Bourdet-Sicard, W. A. Walker, and O. Goulet. 2009. Clinical evidence for immunomodulatory effects of probiotic bacteria. *Journal of Pediatric Gastroenterology and Nutrition* 48 (2): 126–41.

Ruhl, C. E., and J. E. Everhart. 2005. Coffee and tea consumption are associated with a lower incidence of chronic liver disease in the United States. *Gastroenterology* 129 (6): 1928–36.

Saavedra, J. 2000. Probiotics and infectious diarrhea. *American Journal of Gastroenterology* 95 (1 Suppl.): 16–18.

———. 2002. Clinical applications of probiotic agents. *American Journal of Clinical Nutrition* 76 (6): S1147–51.

Salminen, M. K., S. Tynkkynen, H. Rautelin, M. Saxelin, M. Vaara, P. Ruutu, S. Sarna, V. Valtonen, and A. Jarvinen. 2002. *Lactobacillus* bacteremia during a rapid increase in probiotic use of *Lactobacillus rhamnosus* GG in Finland. *Clinical Infectious Diseases* 35: 1155–60.

Scannapieco, F., R. Bush, and S. Paju. 2003. Associations between periodontal disease and risk for atherosclerosis, cardiovascular disease, and stroke. A systematic review. *Annals of Periodontology* 8 (1): 38–53.

Scolapio, J. S., N. Malhi-Chowla, and A. Ukleja. 1999. Nutrition supplementation in patients with acute and chronic pancreatitis. *Gastroenterology Clinics of North America* 28 (3): 695–707.

Selway, S. A. 1990. Potential hazards of long-term acid suppression. *Scandinavian Journal of Gastroenterology* 25 (Suppl. 178): 85–92.

Shaheen, N., and D. F. Ransohoff. 2002. Gastroesophageal reflux, Barrett esophagus, and esophageal cancer: Scientific review. *Journal of the American Medical Association* 287 (15): 1972–81.

Shixian, Q., B. VanCrey, J. Shi, Y. Kakuda, and Y. Jiang. 2007. Green tea extract thermogenesis-induced weight loss by epigallocatechin gallate inhibition of catechol-O-methyltransferase. *Journal of Medicinal Food* 9 (4): 451–58.

Simon, J. A., D. Grady, M. C. Snabes, J. Fong, and D. B. Hunninghake. 1998. Ascorbic acid supplement use and the prevalence of gallbladder disease. Heart and Estrogen-Progestin Replacement Study (HERS) Research Group. *Journal of Clinical Epidemiology* 51 (3): 257–65.

Slattery, M., J. Benson, K. Curtin, K. Ma, D. Schaeffer, and J. Potter. 2000. Carotenoids and colon cancer. *American Journal of Clinical Nutrition* 71 (2): 575–82.

Slattery, M., J. Potter, A. Coates, K. Ma, T. Berry, D. Duncan, and B. Caan. 1997. Plant foods and colon cancer: An assessment of specific foods and their related nutrients (United States). *Cancer Causes and Control* 8 (4): 575–90.

Snowdon, D., M. Gross, and S. Butler. 1996. Antioxidants and reduced functional capacity in the elderly: Findings from the nun study. *The Journals of Gerontology Medical Sciences* 51 (1): M10–16.

Spanier, J. A., C. W. Howden, and M. P. Jones. 2003. A systematic review of alternative therapies in the irritable bowel syndrome. *Archives of Internal Medicine* 163 (3): 265–74.

Spiller, R. 2005. Probiotics: An ideal anti-inflammatory treatment for IBS? *Gastroenterology* 128 (3): 783–85.

Stenson, W. F., D. Cort, J. Rodgers, R. Burakoff, K. DeSchryver-Kecskemeti, T. L. Gramlich, and W. Beeken. 1992. Dietary supplementation with fish oil in ulcerative colitis. *Annals of Internal Medicine* 116 (8): 609–14.

Stewart, W., J. Lieberman, R. Sandler, M. Woods, A. Stemhagen, E. Chee, R. Lipton, and C. Farup. 1999. Epidemiology of constipation (EPOC) study in the United States: Relation of clinical subtypes to sociodemographic features. *American Journal of Gastroenterology* 94 (12): 3530–40.

Stollman, N. H., and J. B. Raskin. 1999. Diagnosis and management of diverticular disease of the colon in adults. Ad Hoc Practice Parameters Committee of the American College of Gastroenterology. *American Journal of Gastroenterology* 94 (11): 3110–21.

Strate, L. L., Y. L. Liu, S. Syngal, W. H. Aldoori, and E. L. Giovannucci. 2008. Nut, corn, and popcorn consumption and the incidence of diverticular disease. *Journal of the American Medical Association* 300 (8): 907–14.

Sullivan, A., and C. E. Nord. 2005. Probiotics and gastrointestinal diseases. *Journal of Internal Medicine* 257 (1): 78–92.

Takahashi, I., and H. Kiyono. 1999. Gut as the largest immunologic tissue. *JPEN: Journal of Parenteral and Enteral Nutrition* 23 (5 Suppl.): 7–12.

Tamboli, C. P., C. Neut, P. Desreumaux, and J. F. Colombel. 2004. Dysbiosis in inflammatory bowel disease. *Gut* 53 (1): 1–4.

Taylor, G. 2001. Bidirectional interrelationships between diabetes and periodontal diseases: An epidemiologic perspective. *Annals of Periodontology* 6: (1): 99–112.

Termanini, B., F. Gibril, V. E. Sutliff, F. Yu, D. J. Venzon, and R. T. Jensen. 1998. Effect of long-term gastric acid suppressive therapy on serum vitamin B12 levels in patients with Zollinger-Ellison syndrome. *American Journal of Medicine* 104 (5): 422–30.

Tuzhilin, S. A., D. A. Dreiling, R. V. Narodetskaja, and L. K. Lukash. 1976. The treatment of patients with gallstones by lecithin. *American Journal of Gastroenterology* 65 (3): 231–35.

Untersmayr, E., I. Scholl, I. Swoboda, W. J. Beil, E. Forster-Waldl, F. Walter, et al. 2003. Antacid medication inhibits digestion of dietary proteins and causes food allergy: A fish allergy model in BALB/c mice. *Journal of Allergy and Clinical Immunology* 112 (3): 616–23.

Upritchard, J., W. Sutherland, and J. Mann. 2000. Effect of supplementation with tomato juice, vitamin E, vitamin C on LDL oxidation and products of inflammatory activity in type 2 diabetes. *Diabetes Care* 23 (6): 733–38.

UpToDate, Inc. http://www.uptodate.com (accessed May 15, 2010).

Vaananen, M., H. Markkanen, V. Tuovinen, A. Kullaa, A. Karinpaa, and E. Kumpusalo. 1993. Periodontal health related to plasma ascorbic acid. *Proceedings of the Finnish Dental Society* 89 (1–2): 51–59.

Vakil, N. 2005. Primary and secondary treatment for *Helicobacter pylori* in the United States. *Reviews in Gastroenterological Disorders* 5 (2): 67–72.

van Poppel, G., D. Verhoeven, H. Verhagen, and R. Goldbohm. 1999. Brassica vegetables and cancer prevention. Epidemiology and mechanisms. *Advances in Experimental Medicine and Biology* 472: 159–68.

Vanderhoof, J. 2000. Probiotics and intestinal inflammatory disorders in infants and children. *Journal of Pediatric Gastroenterology and Nutrition* 30: S34–38.

Vanderpool, C., F. Yan, and D. B. Polk. 2008. Mechanisms of probiotic action: Implications for therapeutic applications in inflammatory bowel diseases. *Inflammatory Bowel Diseases* 14 (11): 1585–96.

Vogelsang, H., P. Ferenci, H. Resch, A. Kiss, and A. Gangl. 1995. Prevention of bone mineral loss in patients with Crohn's disease by long-term oral vitamin D supplementation. *European Journal of Gastroenterology and Hepatology* 7 (7): 609–14.

Waxman, D. 1988. The irritable bowel: A pathological or a psychological syndrome? *Journal of the Royal Society of Medicine* 81 (12): 718–20.

Whorwell, P., L. Altringer, J. Morel, Y. Bond, D. Charbonneau, L. O'Mahony, B. Kiely, F. Shanahan, and E. Quigley. 2007. Efficacy of an encapsulated probiotic *Bifidobacterium infantis* 35624 in women with irritable bowel syndrome. *American Journal of Gastroenterology* 101 (7): 1581–90.

Wilkinson, E., R. Arnold, and K. Folkers. 1976. Bioenergetics in clinical medicine VI. Adjunctive treatment of periodontal disease with coenzyme Q10. *Research Communications in Chemical Pathology and Pharmacology* 14 (4): 715–19.

Wilson, C., T. Rashid, H. Tiwana, H. Beyan, L. Hughes, S. Bansal, A. Ebringer, and A. Binder. 2003. Cytotoxicity responses to peptide antigens in rheumatoid arthritis and ankylosing spondylitis. *Journal of Rheumatology* 30 (5): 972–78.

Wolfe, M. M., D. R. Lichtenstein, and G. Singh. 1999. Gastrointestinal toxicity of nonsteroidal antiinflammatory drugs. *New England Journal of Medicine* 340: 1888–99.

Woolfe, S., E. Kenney, W. Hume, and F. Carranza Jr. 1984. Relationship of ascorbic acid levels of blood and gingival tissue with response to periodontal therapy. *Journal of Clinical Periodontology* 11 (3): 159–65.

Xiao, O. S., Y. Zheng, H. Cai, K. Gu, Z. Chen, W. Zheng, and W. Lu. 2009. Soy food intake and breast cancer survival. *Journal of the American Medical Association* 302 (22): 2437–43.

Young, R. J., and J. A. Vanderhoof. 2004. Two cases of *Lactobacillus* bacteremia during probiotic treatment of short gut syndrome. *Journal of Pediatric Gastroenterology and Nutrition* 39: 436–37.

Zemel, M. B. 2005. The role of dairy foods in weight management. *Journal of the American College of Nutrition* 24 (6): 537S–46S.

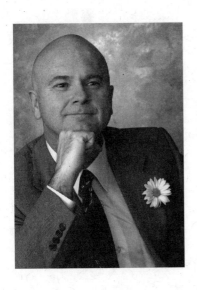

Victor S. Sierpina, MD, is professor of family and integrative medicine at the University of Texas Medical Branch in Galveston, TX, with over thirty years of experience in integrative medicine. His professional practice, courses, and research focus on natural health approaches to disease prevention and wellness.

Foreword writer **David Jones, MD**, is president and director of medical education at the Institute for Functional Medicine in Gig Harbor, WA. He has practiced as a family physician with emphasis in functional and integrative medicine for over thirty years.

Preface writer **Steven G. Pratt, MD, FACS, ABIHM**, is a world-renowned authority on the role of nutrition and lifestyle in the prevention of disease and optimization of health. He is senior staff ophthalmologist at Scripps Memorial Hospital in La Jolla, CA, and author of several books, including *SuperFoods Rx*.

INDEX

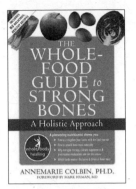
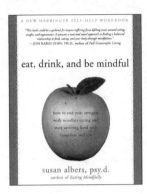
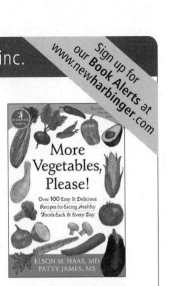
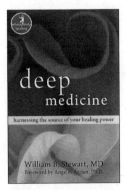
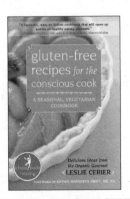
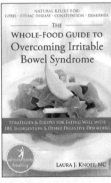